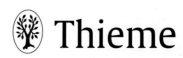

Primary Care Colposcopy

Textbook and Atlas

Erich Burghardt, M. D.
Professor Emeritus and former Chairman
Department of Gynecology and
Obstetrics
University of Graz
Austria

Hellmuth Pickel, M. D.
Professor
Department of Gynecology
and Obstetrics
University of Graz
Austria

Frank Girardi, M. D.
Head of Department
of Gynecology and obstetrics
Thermenklinikum
Baden, Austria

With the collaboration of

Karl Tamussino, M.D.
Professor
Department of Gynecology
and Obstetrics
University of Graz
Austria

322 illustrations, most in color
11 tables

Thieme
Stuttgart · New York

Library of Congress Cataloging-in-Publication Data
is available from the publisher

This book represents selections from the third edition of E. Burghardt's **Colposcopy** – Cervical Pathology, published and copyrighted 1998 by Georg Thieme Verlag, Stuttgart, Germany.

© 2004 Georg Thieme Verlag, Rüdigerstrasse 14,
D-70469 Stuttgart, Germany
http://www.thieme.de
Thieme New York, 333 Seventh Avenue,
New York, NY 10001, USA
http://www.thieme.com

Typesetting by primustype Hurler GmbH, Notzingen
Printed in Germany by Grammlich, Pliezhausen

ISBN 3-13-130721-8 (GTV)
ISBN 1-58890-092-4 (TNY)   1 2 3 4 5

Important Note: Medicine is an ever-changing science udergoing continual development. Research and clinical experience are continually expanding our knowledge, in particular our knowledge of proper treatment and drug therapy. Insofar as this book mentions any dosage or application, readers may rest assured that the authors, editors, and publishers have made every effort to ensure that such references are in accordance with **the state of knowledge at the time of production of the book.**

Nevertheless, this does not involve, imply, or express any guarantee or responsibility on the part of the publishers with respect of any dosage instructions and forms of application stated in the book. **Every user is requested to examine carefully** the manufacturer's leaflets accompanying each drug and to check, if necessary in consultation with a physician or specialist, whether the dosage schedules mentioned therein or the contraindications stated by the manufacturer differ from the statements made in the present book. Such examination is particularly important with drugs that are either rarely used or have been newly released on the market. Every dosage schedule or every form of application used is entirely at the user's risk and responsibility. The authors and publishers request every user to report to the publishers any discrepancies or inaccuracies noticed.

Some of the product names, patents, and registered designs referred to in this book are in fact registered trademarks or proprietary names, even though specific reference to this fact is not always made in the text. Therefore, the appearance of a name without a designation as proprietary is not to be construed as a representation by the publisher that it is in the public domain.

Preface

Colposcopy is an accepted and widely used technique to examine the lower genital tract. The number of textbooks on colposcopy testifies to the rapid development of the technique over the last 20 years. The first edition of this book came out in German in 1984 (1). Since then revised editions have appeared in Spanish, Japanese, French, Italian as well as English (2).

The present edition is a compact, user-oriented resource for general practioners, nurses, and other nonspecialists. Accordingly we have left out detailed histologic pictures and descriptions while keeping the colposcopic images that are the backbone of the book. So-called "extended colposcopy" (i.e., with the acetic acid and the iodine test) has been given ample coverage. We emphasize how to assess the abnormal vascular patterns that frequently signal underlying problems that require treatment. Like its predecessors this book intends to explain both the fundamentals of colposcopic technique as well as how colposcopy can help appreciate the dynamic processes at the cervix that we have to understand to prevent invasive cervical cancer.

E. Burghardt

Contents

Introduction

Colposcopy

Hinselmann introduced colposcopy as a method for early detection of cervical cancer in 1924 (5), long before cervical cytology was developed. The goal of both colposcopy and cytology is to predict the histologic status of the cervix. A number of studies have shown that using colposcopy and cytology together increases diagnostic accuracy (1). However, colposcopy is often limited to patients with abnormal cervical cytology and has not achieved worldwide acceptance as a screening modality. In this setting, the goal of colposcopy is to visualize abnormal areas on the cervix, and to identify the most severe area for directed biopsy. It is important to appreciate that colposcopy cannot provide a histologic diagnosis. This requires a tissue specimen. Predicting the histology of original squamous epithelium, ectopy, or completely normal transformation zones is relatively easy. Predicting the histology of abnormal colposcopic findings, some of which differ only in subtle features, is more difficult. Unfortunately, no colposcopic features are pathognomonic of malignancy.

We use the current colposcopic terminology presented at the World Congress for Colposcopy and Cervical Pathology in Barcelona in 2002 (Table 1) (13). The subclassification of white epithelium, mosaic, punctation, and leukoplakia into major and minor categories implies a certain qualitative assessment. We use the term *atypical transformation zone* interchangeably with *white epithelium*. It is also important to remember that this modification was meant to apply to colposcopy used as a screening test in all women, not just to evaluate those with abnormal cervical cytology reports.

In practice, the colposcopist has to distinguish between non-suspicious and suspicious findings, and he or she is increasingly able to do so once experience is gained. Suspicious findings are not always synonymous with abnormal findings because the latter are not always due to premalignant or invasive lesions.

Cytology

The idea of evaluating of *cytological* material from the cervix and vagina for the diagnosis of cervical carcinoma and its precursors is the achievement of *George N. Papanicolaou*. Papanicolaou himself developed the first system of cytologic reporting or classifying of cervical cytology in 1954 (7). This system graded cytologic specimens from I to V according to the presence and severity of cytological abnormalities. In 1953 *Reagan* et al.(8) proposed a terminology that could be used for cytology and histology. The term „carcinoma in situ“ was suggested for cytologic and histologic abnormalities associated with a true neoplastic lesion, and the term „dysplasia“ for cytologic abnormalities associated with a better differentiated lesion. The pre-cancerous potential of the latter was unknown. It was proposed to divide dysplasia into mild, moderate and severe forms.

The *Richart* (9) classification (1967) was initially a histologic classification. Later it was applied to cytology and was adopted by the WHO in 1973 (10). The term „cervical intra-epithelial neoplasia“ (CIN) was introduced to replace the terms dysplasia and carcinoma in situ. The main objective of this classification was to define a morphologic and biologic continuum between dysplastic lesions and carcinoma in situ, leading to the concept that all these lesions, including CIN I, were pre-cancerous. Because it is hard to distinguish between severe dysplasia and carcinoma in situ, this classification combined the two entities under the term CIN III. Until 1988, most cytology laboratories used one of these three classifications, Papanicolaou, dysplasia-carcinoma in situ, or the CIN-terminology.

The current terminology for cervical cytology, *The Bethesda System (TBS)*, was developed by a panel convened in 1988 under the auspices of the National Cancer Institute. The system was revised in 1991 and 2001 (6, 12). TBS replaced three levels of CIN with two levels: low- and high-grade squamous intraepithelial lesions (LSIL and HSIL). The category of benign cellular changes was eliminated in 2001. Instead, these smears were shifted to either the negative category (no evidence of intraepithelial lesion) or the *atypical* squamous cells category. The category of ASCUS (atypical cells of undetermined significance) in the 1991 Bethesda System was subjective, poorly reproducible and overutilized and this category was eliminated in 2001. Smears that were not negative but did not meet the criteria for SIL would be called atypical squamous cells (ASC) and would be subclassified either as of undetermined significance (ASCUS) or as suggestive of a high-grade SIL (ASC-H) (13).

The classification of abnormalities of the columnar (glandular) epithelium in TBS 1991 has been more problematic. Glandular abnormalities were divided into three general categories: cytologically benign endometrial cells in a postmenopausal woman, atypical glandular cells of undetermined significance (AGUS), and adenocarcinoma. AGUS was divided into AGUS favoring a reactive process (AUGS-FN), and AGUS not otherwise specified (AGUS-NOS). Whenever possible, adenocarcinoma was classified based on its cell of origin. In 2001 the Bethesda panel concluded that AGUS-FN was clearly a different and distinguishable cytologic entity that probably represents adenocarcinoma in situ of the endocervix. The criteria for adenocarcinoma in situ have been shown to be predictive and reproducible and it was recommended that a separate category should be established for these findings. Further it was felt that the term AGUS-FR did not always reflect the potential seriousness of the underlying condition, and this term was eliminated. This left only those smears in which the atypical glandular cells were truly of undetermined significance to be called atypical glandular cells (AGC). Qualifying statements are added to AGC to indicate cellular origin of the atypical cells (endocervical, endometrial, or glandular-NOS) (13).

Human papillomavirus infection

The etiologic relationship of HPV to cervical cancer is firmly established. The current list of cancer-associated HPV-types includes four high-risk types (types 16, 18, 31, and 45) and nine intermediate-risk types (types 33, 35, 39, 51, 52, 56, 58, 59 and 68). Seventy-five percent of cervical cancers are infected with type 16, 18, 31, or 45 (4). HPV infections are initiated when the virus gains access to basal cells of an epithelial surface through minor trauma or sexual intercourse. HPV 16 is the predominant type in squamous cancers, HPV 18 the predominant type in adenocarcinomas. Infections with multiple subtypes occur in 2 % to 20 % of women, and these women are at increased risk of developing CIN or SIL compared with women infected with a single type (4).

Subclinical HPV infections may be 10 to 30 times more common than cytologically apparent infections. Most cervical HPV infections are transient (3).

Women with borderline and low-grade abnormalities on cervical cytology have a risk for progression to invasive cervical cancer over 24 month of 1 to 2 per 1000 women without treatment. High viral load and persistent HPV infection may be risk factors for high-grade cytologic abnormalities (11).

References

1. Burghardt E. Kolposkopie. Spezielle Zervixpathologie. Lehrbuch und Atlas. Thieme. Stuttgart, 1984.
2. Burghardt E, Pickel H, Girardi F. Colposcopy – cervical pathology. Textbook and Atlas. 3rd edition. Thieme. Stuttgart, 1998
3. Castle PE, Wacholder S, Sherman ME, Lorincz AT, Glass AG, Scott DR, Rush BB, Demuth F, Schiffman M. Absolute risk of a subsequent abnormal Pap among oncogenic human papillomavirus DNA-positive, cytologically negative women. Cancer 95:2145, 2002
4. Clifford GM, Smith JS, Plummer M, Munoz N, Franceschi S. Human papillomavirus types in invasive cervical cancer worldwide: a meta-analysis. Cancer, 88:63–73, 2003
5. Hinselmann H. Verbesserung der Inspektionsmöglichkeit der Vulva, Vagina und Portio. Münch Med Wschr 77:1733 ff, 1925
6. O'Meara AT: Present standards for cervical cancer screening. Curr Opin Oncol 14:505–511, 2002
7. Papanicolaou GN: Atlas of exfoliative cytology. The Commonwealth Fund, Cambridge 1954
8. Reagan JW, Seidemann IL, Saracusa Y: The cellular morphology of carcinoma in situ and dysplasia or atypical hyperplasia of the uterine cervix. Cancer, 6:224–235, 1953
9. Richart RM: Natural history of cervical intraepithelial neoplasia. Clin Obstet Gynec 10:748–794, 1967
10. Riotton G, Christopherson WM: Cytology of the female genital tract. World Health Organization, Geneva 1973
11. Schlecht NF, Trevisan A, Duarte-Franco E, Rohan TE, Ferenczy A, Villa LL, Franco EL. Viral load as a predictor of the risk of cervical intraepithelial neoplasia. Int J Cancer 103:519–524, 2003
12. Spitzer M, Johnson C. Terminology in cervical cytology: The Bethesda System. In Apgar BS, Brothman GL, Spither M. Colposcopy principles and practice. An integrated textbook and atlas. Saunders Philadelphia, 2002.
13. Walker P, Dexeus S, De Palo G, Barrasso R, Campion M, Girardi F, Jakob C, Roy M. International terminology of colposcopy: an updated report from the International Federation for Cervical Pathology and Colposcopy. Obstet Gynecol 101:175–177, 2003

Table 1 International Federation of Cervical Pathology and Colposcopy Colposcopic Classification

I	**Normal colposcopic findings**
	Original squamous epithelium
	Columnar epithelium
	Transformation zone
II	**Abnormal colposcopic findings**
	Flat acetowhite epithelium
	Dense acetowhite epithelium*
	Fine mosaic
	Coarse mosaic*
	Fine punctation
	Coarse punctation*
	Iodine partial positivity
	Iodine negativity*
	Atypical vessels*
III	**Colposcopic features suggestive of invasive cancer**
IV	**Unsatisfactory colposcopy**
	Squamocolumnar junction not visible
	Severe inflammation, severe atrophy, trauma
	Cervix not visible
V	**Miscellaneous findings**
	Condylomata
	Keratosis
	Erosion
	Inflammation
	Atrophy
	Deciduosis
	Polyps

* Major changes.

1

The Colposcope

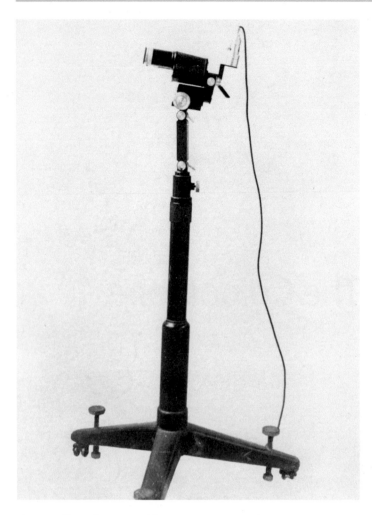

Fig. 1.**1** First colposcope with a fixed mount, by Leitz. This model was used by Hinselmann

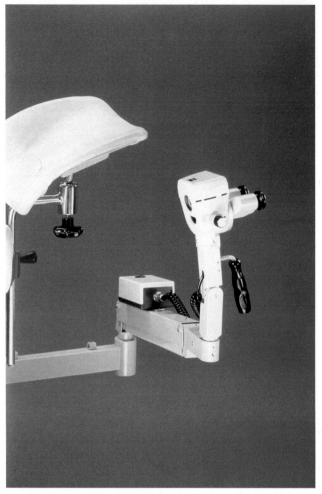

Fig. 1.**2** Chair-mounted colposcope with an integrated lamp and fixed ×5 or ×3, ×5 and ×8 magnifications (Colposcope E, Carl Zeiss, Oberkochen, Germany)

Hinselmann used Leitz lenses mounted on a pile of books for his first colposcopic examination (1). An ordinary lamp normally used for gynecologic examination was the light source; when placed above the operator's head, it illuminated the cervix. The first colposcope was a fixed binocular instrument mounted on a tripod and equipped with a light source and a mirror to center the light (Fig. 1.**1**).

Modern colposcopes permit magnification between ×6 and ×40. A ×10 times enlargement is most suitable for routine use. Higher magnification reveals minor features, but is not necessary for accurate diagnosis. The colposcope should be equipped with a *green filter* that can be easily swung into position: it filters out red and thereby enhances the vascular appearance by making the vessels dark.

The colposcope can be mounted in different ways. For routine use, a swivel arm attached to the examination table is most suitable (Fig. 1.**2**). It can be easily adjusted by hand in both vertical and horizontal directions. The mobile but mounted colposcope is independent of the examination table

and can be moved from place to place (Fig. 1.**3**). It can be fitted with a swivel arm and, when the wheels are locked, can be used in the same way as the examination-table mounted model. Colposcopes mounted on the wall are easy to handle on account of their mobility (Fig. 1.**5**). The head of the instrument may be tilted up, down and sideways. There is usually no need for the fine adjustment, as a sharp focus can be achieved just as easily by positioning the instrument at the right working distance of 20 to 24 cm.

The most important accessories are the photographic and video equipment (Fig. 2.**2**) and the teaching arm (Fig. 1.**4**). Colpophotography is described in more detail elsewhere (see p. 142, Documentation of Colposcopic Findings). The teaching arm is an invaluable aid. Although only monocular, it offers the student instruction by an experienced colposcopist that no atlas can replace (see Fig. 2.**1**).

Simple low-power instruments without any accessories (Fig. 1.**5**) as well as sophisticated ones with an electrically operated zoom lens and fine adjustment and camera (Fig. 1.**3**)

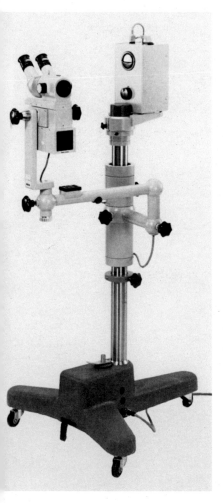

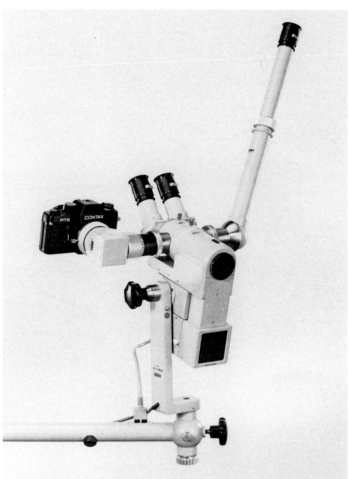

Fig. 1.**3** Colposcope mounted on a stand (OPMI 1H, Carl Zeiss, Oberkochen, Germany). This model has five magnifications and fine power

Fig. 1.**4** Colposcope on a swivel arm (OPMI 6 SH, Carl Zeiss, Oberkochen, Germany). This model has zoom magnification and power fine focus

are available. Prices vary accordingly. For routine use, a simple colposcope is quite adequate, but for teaching both a camera and video equipment or a teaching arm are mandatory (Figs. 1.**4**, 2.**2**).

Reference

1 Hinselmann H. Die Ätiologie, Symptomatologie und Diagnostik des Uteruscarcinoms. In: Veit J, Stöckel W, eds. Handbuch der Gynäkologie, vol. 6:1. Munich: Bergmann, 1930:854.

2

Colposcopic Training

For effective colposcopy, as for any endoscopic method, the student must become familiar with the instruments and the technique of the examination. Then he or she can learn to appreciate colposcopic findings in the vulva, vagina and cervix.

Instruments and Technique

As discussed in Chapter 1, the colposcope is a simple instrument, the handling of which should pose no difficulties, even for beginners. The eyepieces are adjusted individually. The instrument is focused by moving the swivel arm to the working distance for the particular scope. It is usually unnecessary to use the fine focus. The built-in light source provides excellent illumination.

For practice, the student can examine familiar objects such as his hand, small print, or a coin, as with a magnifying glass. The various color filters and enlargements can be tried out.

The beginner commonly uses too high magnification. For routine work, magnification of ×10 is quite adequate. Higher magnification is needed only to study details. Smaller enlargements can be used for panoramic photographs.

Colpophotography is simple and produces high-quality pictures. The cervix has to be exposed well and the camera focused correctly (see Chapter 11).

Understanding Colposcopic Findings

Basic knowledge of colposcopic theory and an appreciation of cervical pathology are essential. Only by correlating colposcopic and histologic changes can the colposcopic findings be interpreted correctly (see Chapter 10). Connections must be drawn among the various colposcopic appearances to formulate a concept of the physiologic and pathologic processes that take place at the cervix.

It is best to take a biopsy of colposcopically suspicious lesions as soon as they are detected rather than wait for the results of exfoliative cytology. If the aim is to reduce the number of biopsies, one can wait for the cytology result and obtain another smear if it is normal. Under no circumstances should a colposcopically suspect but cytologically negative lesion be ignored.

Application of the Equipment

Once a working knowledge of colposcopic appearances has been acquired from a well-illustrated textbook or teaching slides, it is very helpful for the student to work with an experienced colposcopist who can demonstrate and explain findings step-by-step. This can be done with a teaching arm (Fig. 2.1) or video equipment (Fig. 2.2). A color video camera can record part or all of the examination. Obtaining a biopsy should be demonstrated and then practiced. Video monitoring also lets the patient watch the examination. The results of a randomized trial showed that video colposcopy increased patient satisfaction with preventive health care (1). Video ap-

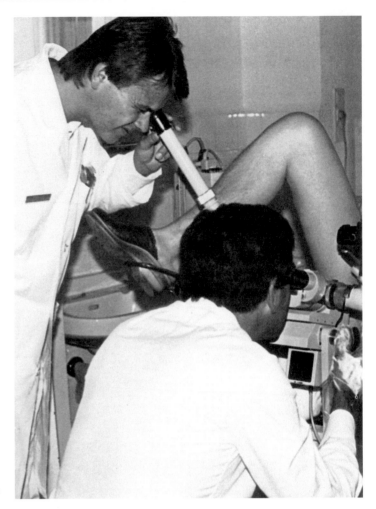

Fig. 2.**1**   Colposcope with a teaching arm

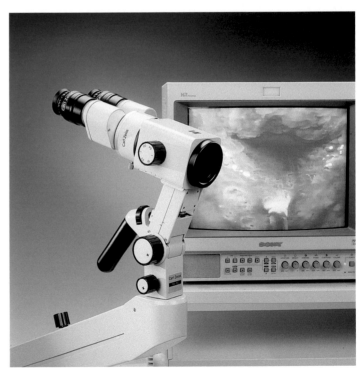

Fig. 2.**2**   Videocolposcopy

plications for teaching and documentation will undoubtedly increase as the technology advances.

The already practicing physician, for whom this kind of training is impractical, is advised to study the theoretical aspects. Courses are available at entry and advanced levels where individual problems can be discussed with the faculty.

Further improvement takes practice. The time it takes to improve and the degree of competence attained depend on how the colposcope is used. Ideally, colposcopy should be an integral part of every gynecologic examination. This is also a convenient way to gain experience and will soon convince the practitioner that the method is not as costly and time-consuming as often stated. With repeated colposcopy, the practitioner will feel uncomfortable performing a speculum examination without a colposcope.

This approach will expedite the recognition of benign findings and pave the way for understanding the dynamics of the events at the cervix, which, if they take a wrong turn, can lead to atypia. The beginner is advised to start with the study of ectopy and continue with the protean manifestations of the transformation zone. Only by becoming familiar with these benign findings can one recognize those that are no longer benign.

Certain colposcopic findings are easy to categorize as benign or highly suspicious. But in between there is a wide spectrum of appearances that are difficult to appraise (see Chapter 9). The same applies to cytology. The degree of uncertainty depends on the experience of the examiner. Obtaining a biopsy of every doubtful finding accelerates the learning process and avoids serious mistakes. By correlating the colposcopic appearance with the histologic findings, the practitioner will gain confidence and the number of biopsies will decrease. The chance of missing a significant finding is considerably reduced by concomitant cytology.

Reference

1 Greimel ER, Gappmayer-Löcker E, Girardi F, Huber HP. Increasing women's knowledge and satisfaction with cervical cancer screening. J Psychosomat Obstet Gynaecol 1997; 18:273.

3

Colposcopic Instruments

3.1

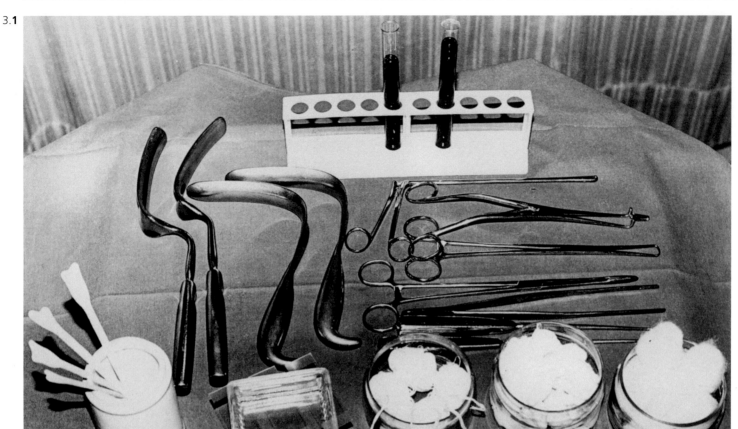

3.2

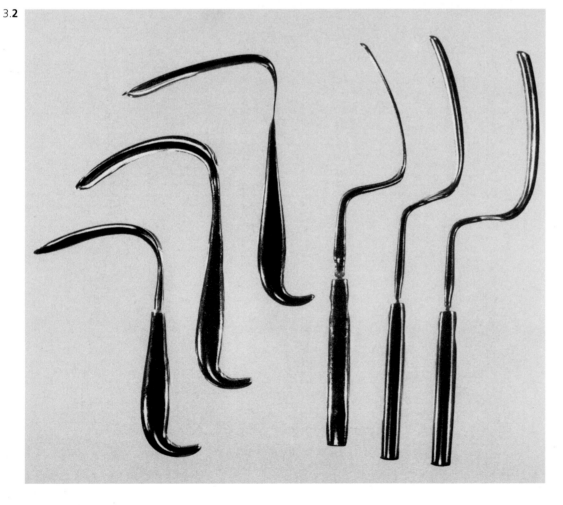

Fig. 3.**1** **Instruments for colposcopy:** specula, anatomic forceps, tenacula, endocervical speculum, and biopsy instruments: *above,* iodine solution in test tubes; *below,* swabs, tampons, and utensils for obtaining and fixing cytology smears

Fig. 3.**2** **Vaginal retractors of various sizes,** with the back blades on the left and front blades on the right

The instruments needed for colposcopy are few and not expensive. In addition to the colposcope, one needs retractors, biopsy instruments, an endocervical speculum, anatomic forceps, tenacula, and swabs (Fig. 3.**1**).

Specula

Vaginal retractors (Fig. 3.**2**) or a duckbill speculum (Fig. 3.**3**) can be used. The retractors provide a clear view of the vagina. A disadvantage is that the front blade needs to be held by an assistant, but the assistant can expedite the examination by passing instruments and swabs (see Fig. 5.**1**). The self-retaining duckbill speculum has the advantage that it can be manipulated by the colposcopist alone (see Fig. 5.**2**). Because of the different capacity of the vagina, specula of various types and sizes may have to be used.

Forceps

Anatomic forceps (Fig. 3.**4**, left) at least 20 cm long are needed to hold dry and moist swabs. They are more practical than tenacula.

Endocervical Speculum

The endocervical speculum (Fig. 3.**4**), or similar instruments, allow inspection of the endocervical canal and are most useful in multiparous patients. Ideally, the distal dilating jaws should be able to be displaced laterally from the remaining shaft of the instrument so that visibility is not obscured when the instrument is introduced into the canal.

Fig. 3.**3** **Duckbill specula** of various calibers

Fig. 3.**4** **Anatomic forceps (left) and endocervical speculum (right)**; the latter allows better exposure of the endocervical canal

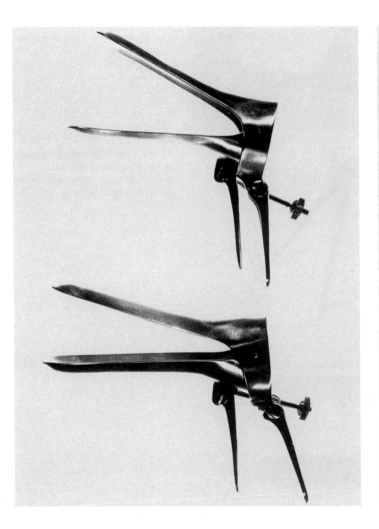

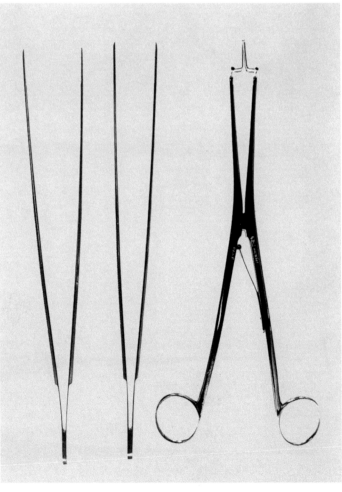

Containers

Swabs are stored in sterilized metal cylinders. For the examination, they are placed in a bowl from which they can be easily retrieved with forceps. For the acetic acid test (see p. 20) swabs are soaked in 3% acetic acid and handled with forceps. Lugol's solution (see p. 23) is put into test tubes, which are placed in a rack. Tampons, which can be removed by the patient later (Fig. 3.**5**), can be kept in a sterilizable metal container.

Biopsy Instruments

There are several types of biopsy instruments (Fig. 3.**6**). They are usually pistol-shaped, and have a scissors-like action, with shafts measuring between 20 and 25 cm.

Sharp curettes of various sizes are needed for scraping the endocervical canal and to obtain material from clinically invasive cancers. To curet a narrow endocervical canal, instruments with fine, sharp grooves are more practical than spoon-shaped ones.

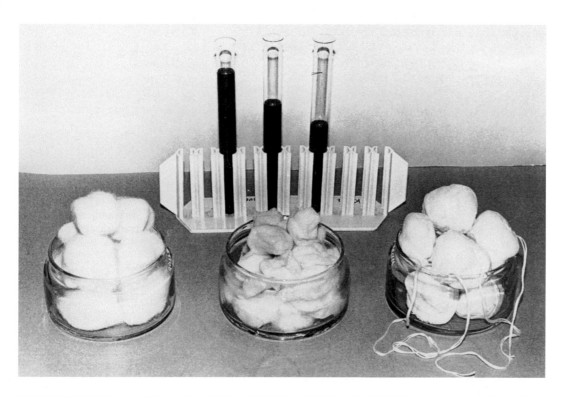

Fig. 3.**5** **Iodine solution in test tubes:** far left, dry cotton-wool swabs; middle, cotton-wool swabs saturated with acetic acid; right, tampons with strings used to stop bleeding after biopsy

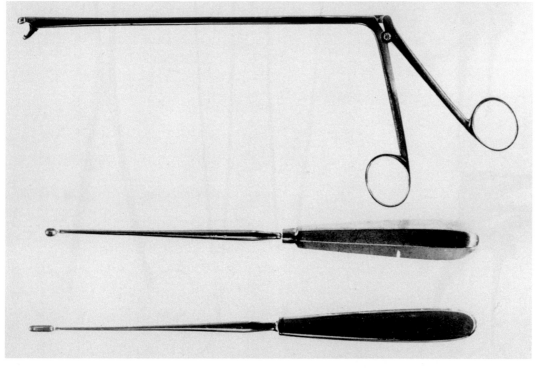

Fig. 3.**6** **Punch biopsy forceps, sharp spoon-shaped and grooved biopsy instruments for endocervical curettage** (from top to bottom)

Tenacula

To prevent slipping of the biopsy punch and to obtain a truly directed biopsy, fixation of the cervix is sometimes necessary. The cervix is easily and painlessly held with a single-toothed tenaculum (Fig. 3.**7**). Cervical polyps can be avulsed easily with polyp forceps (Fig. 3.**7**).

Chrobak's Sound

Chrobak's sound (Fig. 3.**8**) is useful to distinguish between invasive carcinomas and papillomas or flat ectocervical ulcers (see p. 78). It is a thin probe with a bulbous head. In contact with normal tissue or benign tumors, it encounters an elastic resistance; however, it sinks into soft malignant tissue as into butter.

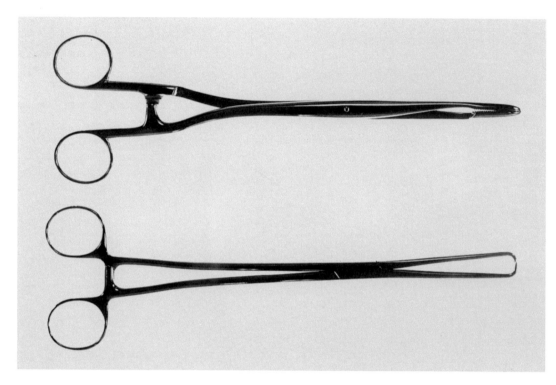

Fig. 3.**7**   **Polyp forceps and single-toothed tenaculum**

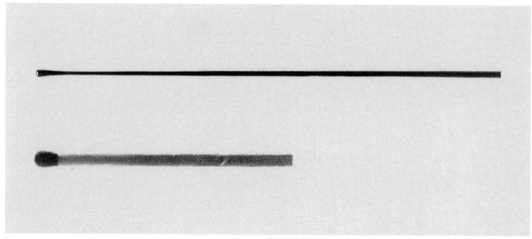

Fig. 3.**8**   **Chrobak's sound**

4

Special
Colposcopic
Techniques

The acetic acid test and the iodine test (Schiller test), as well as the use of the green filter, can all be traced back to Hinselmann. They are still integral parts of the colposcopic examination. A host of other techniques have been suggested for specific problem areas.

Acetic Acid Test

Hinselmann used a 3% solution of acetic acid mainly to get rid of mucus (3, 4). After removing vaginal secretions with dry swabs (see Chapter 5), the cervical epithelium is still masked to some extent by a film of mucus, especially in the presence of ectopy. Cleansing the cervix (see p. 33) with acetic acid enhances the colposcopic features. This applies especially to the grape-like structure of columnar epithelium in ectopy. However, all epithelial lesions become more distinct: the color changes are accentuated, and the various structures become more easily distinguishable from each other (Fig. 4.**1a, b**).

Ectopy shows a distinct color change after application of acetic acid. The intense dark red ectopic columnar epithelium becomes paler and displays shades of pink to white. At the same time, the grape-like structures become more pronounced because of swelling and enlargement of the villi. The acetic acid therefore not only affects the mucus, but also interacts with certain epithelia, making them swell and change their color (Fig. 4.**2a, b**).

Similar changes can be seen in altered epithelia, as described by Burghardt in 1959 (1) in connection with the definition of the *atypical transformation zone*. The epithelial swelling caused by acetic acid turns atypical epithelium white and ac-

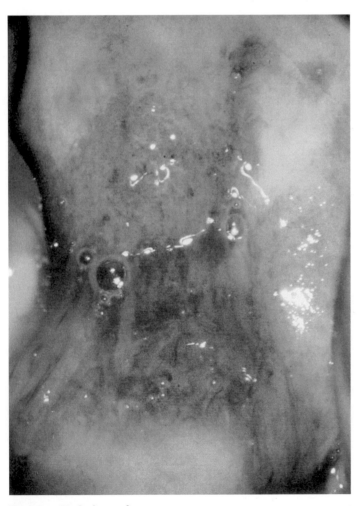

Fig. 4.**1a   Typical transformation zone** before application of acetic acid. The fine details are clouded by mucus

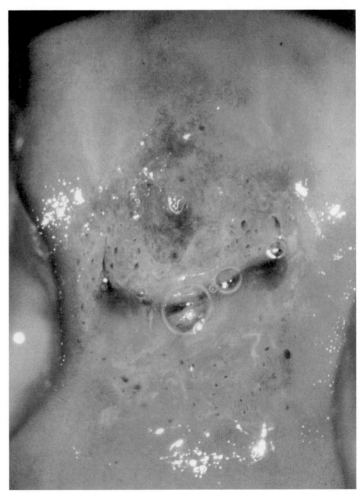

Fig. 4.**1b   Removal of the mucus after acetic acid** reveals the transformation zone with its gland openings

centuates its surface contour (Fig. 4.**3a, b**). The patterns of mosaic and punctation also become more distinct, and the red partitions or the fine petechiae stand out against the white epithelium (Fig. 4.**4a, b**).

Because the effect on pathologic epithelium is not as rapid as on ectopic columnar epithelium, the white epithelium that appears after application of acetic acid should not be confused with leukoplakia. Occasionally, however, poorly keratinized surface lesions will become visible only after cleansing with acetic acid, when they immediately change from pale white to gray, do not undergo swelling, and do not change with time.

Acetic acid therefore plays a decisive role in colposcopic diagnosis (see Chapter 5). No colposcopic examination is complete without it.

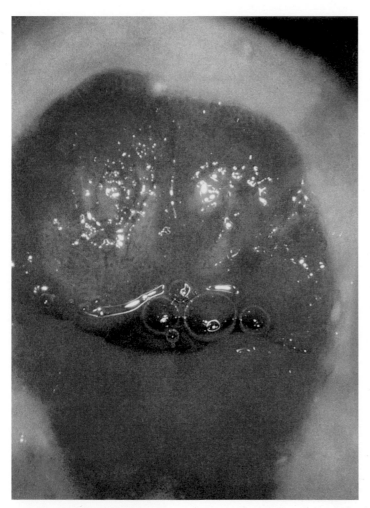

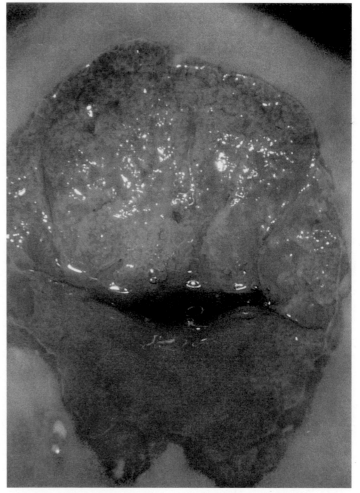

Fig. 4.**2a**   **Large, intensely red area around the external os.**
The border with the normal squamous epithelium seems abrupt. The lesion apparently extends into the cervical canal

Fig. 4.**2b**   **Application of acetic acid evokes the grape-like structure of the mucosa covered by columnar epithelium.** Note the blanching of the previously intensely red area caused by the swelling of the columnar epithelium. In the adjacent squamous epithelium on the posterior lip of the cervix, individual gland openings indicate that transformation has occurred

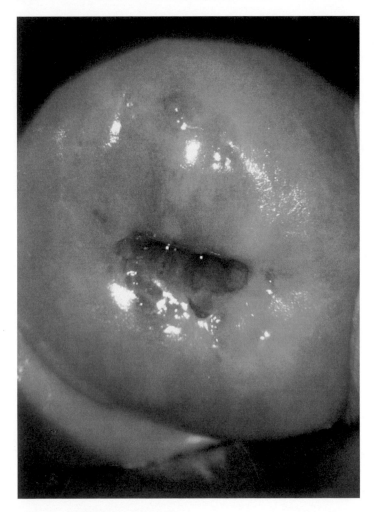

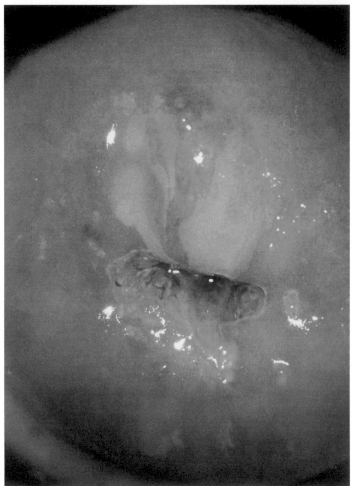

Fig. 4.**3 a**   **An indistinct red area on the anterior lip of the external os.** On the posterior lip there is a small, intensely red area

Fig. 4.**3 b**   Application of acetic acid reveals a number of sharply demarcated white areas on the anterior lip. There are some cuffed gland openings near the white areas. Histology showed CIN 2 (H-SIL). The area on the posterior lip is columnar epithelium with a narrow transformation zone on the edge of it

Fig. 4.**4 a**   **Before the applica-** ▷ **tion of acetic acid, the transformation zone is inconspicuous.** Only the experienced colposcopist will detect an early lesion at the 12-o'clock position, outside the transformation zone

Fig. 4.**4 b**   The white color and mosaic pattern of CIN 3 (H-SIL) are due to cellular edema caused by acetic acid

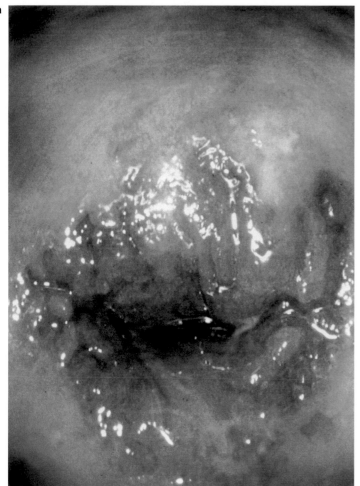
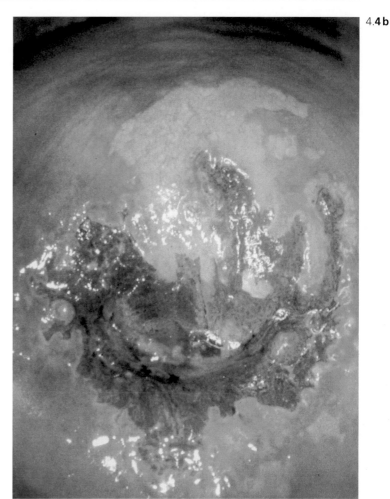

Schiller (Iodine) Test

The rapid action of iodine and its special significance make it an important diagnostic aid for assessing colposcopic findings.

Lugol's iodine solution was first used in clinical diagnosis by Schiller in 1929 (6) and ever since (4, 5, 7–14). Unfortunately, the value of the Schiller test is being debated. Some eminent colposcopists do not use it or do not refer to it, which is also unfortunate because it can yield important additional information for the evaluation of colposcopic morphology. The 1% iodine solution consists of 2 g iodine and 4 g potassium iodide dissolved in 200 ml distilled water.

The *Schiller* test depends on the interaction between iodine and glycogen. The glycogen-containing vaginal epithelium of women of reproductive age takes up iodine to produce an intense mahogany brown. Glycogen-free epithelium does not stain with iodine (Fig. 4.**5**). Such an area is referred to as *iodine negative.*

1. Iodine solution stains normal glycogen-containing squamous epithelium uniformly deep brown. Such epithelium is found during the reproductive period and reflects the influence of estrogens (Fig. 4.**5**).

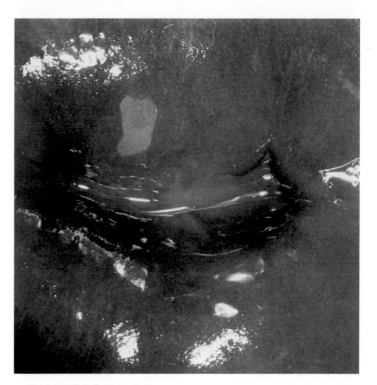

Fig. 4.**5** **Original squamous epithelium** displays uniform mahogany staining with iodine. Note a sharply demarcated iodine-negative area at the 11-o'clock position, referred to as Schiller-positive

2. Columnar epithelium does not stain with iodine (Fig. 4.6) nor does thin regenerating epithelium, seen during the early stages of squamous metaplasia or ascending healing (Fig. 4.7). Failure to stain with iodine is useful to assess inflammatory lesions, which, because of their increased vascularity and capillary dilatation, can mimic punctation. But their margins are indistinct and do not react significantly with iodine (Fig. 4.8a, b).

3. Developing atypical epithelium stains with iodine as described below (5) even while still thin. This is an important difference between the normal and the atypical transformation zone.

4. A colposcopic lesion, as well as the whole length of the vagina, can display all shades between tan and the chestnut brown of normal squamous epithelium (Fig. 4.9). The vagina can have a stippled brown appearance, especially after menopause, when the effect of estrogen wanes. The postmenopausal cervix and vagina stain light brown to yellow (Figs. 4.10 and 7.3).

The various shades of brown of the *normal transformation zone* depend on the *maturity*, that is, the glycogen content, of the squamous epithelium (Fig. 4.11). The squamous epithelium in the fully developed transformation zone stains mahogany brown. The transformation zone in such cases can be recognized only by the gland openings and the retention cysts (Fig. 4.12a, b). The deep-brown color distinguishes it from the atypical transformation zone, as atypical and acanthotic epithelia are almost always glycogen-free.

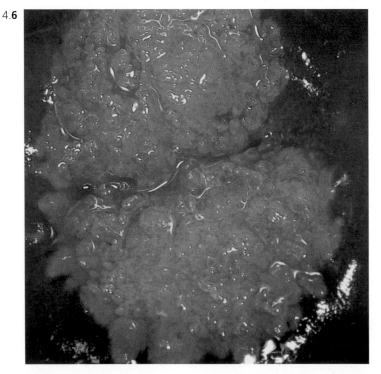

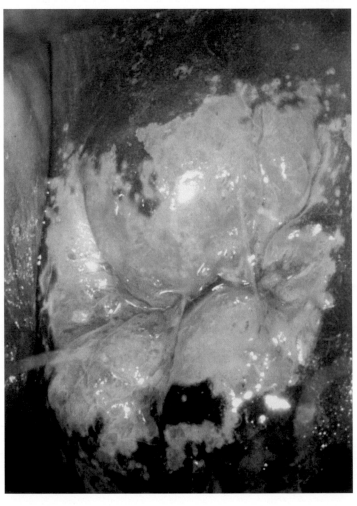

4.6

4.7

Fig. 4.**6**   **The columnar epithelium of an ectopy does not stain with iodine.** It shows only a slight discoloration due to the thin film of solution veiling it. The original epithelium stains characteristically deep brown

Fig. 4.**7**   **The typical transformation zone does not stain with iodine.** Note the contrast with the mahogany color of original squamous epithelium

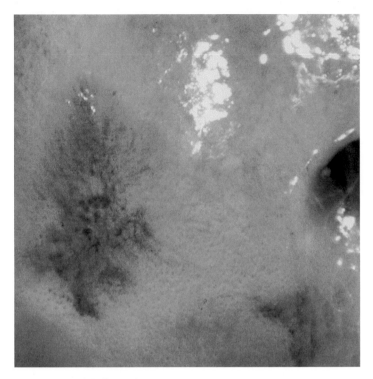

Fig. 4.**8 a   Red, inflamed area**
lateral to the external os

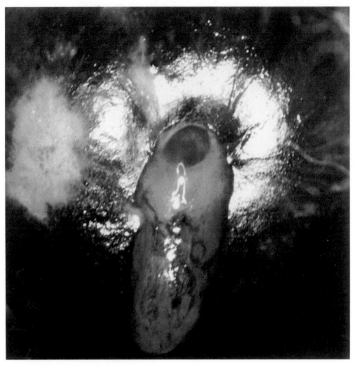

Fig. 4.**8 b   This area does not
stain with iodine,** and is poorly
demarcated from the adjacent
deep-brown original epithelium

4.**9**

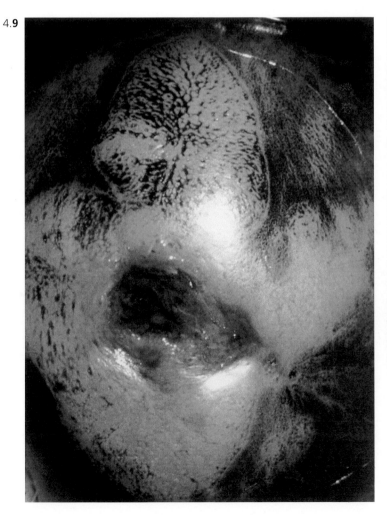

4.**10**

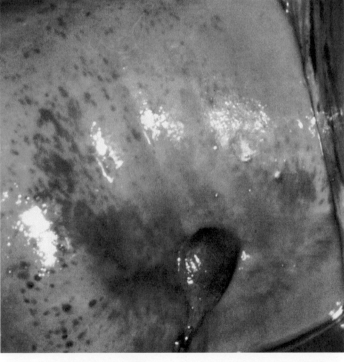

Fig. 4.**9   This transformation
zone has a stippled appearance
with iodine,** due to the various
stages of development of the
metaplastic epithelium

Fig. 4.**10   Yellowish light-brown
of atrophic epithelium after
iodine staining.** At least some of
the dark spots are due to subepithelial hemorrhages

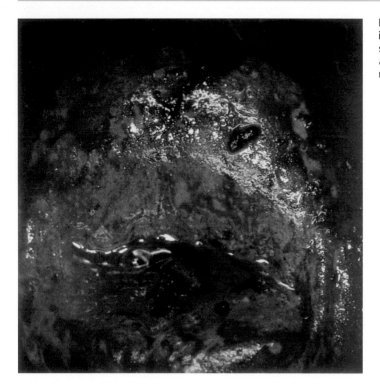

Fig. 4.**11**   **When transformation is more advanced, various shades of brown may appear,** according to the maturity of the metaplastic epithelium

Fig. 4.**12a**   **Very different appearance of the transformation zones of the two lips.** On the anterior lip, the squamous epithelium is attenuated over re- tention cysts, and blood vessels course over their surfaces. The posterior lip shows acetowhite epithelium and gland openings

Fig. 4.**12b**   **Surprising reaction with iodine.** The epithelium covering the retention cyst is fully mature and contains glycogen. The area on the posterior lip, which stains partly yellow or not at all with iodine, was carcinoma in situ (CIN 3, H-SIL) histologically

4.**12a**

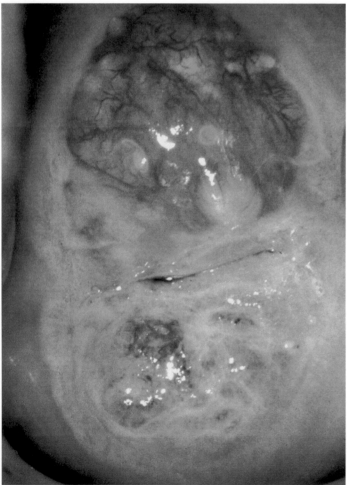

4.**12b**

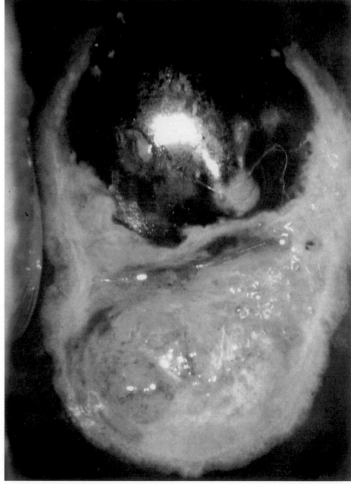

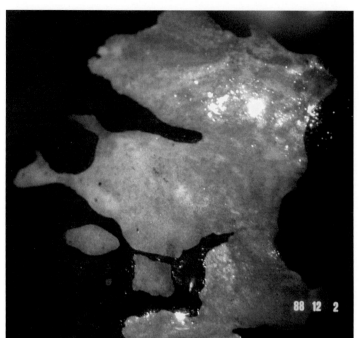

5. Iodine solution reacts with colposcopic lesions to produce a characteristic canary yellow, especially when due to *acanthotic or atypical epithelia* (Figs. 4.**13**–4.**16**) that are glycogen-free. Large transformation zones can become distinctly yellow, in which case the designation *atypical transformation zone* can be used. In some cases, only portions of the transformation zone stain yellow (Fig. 4.**16**). Such areas should be regarded with suspicion, should be carefully searched for, and should always be biopsied.

Fig. 4.**13** **Nonsuspicious iodine-yellow area.** The lesion is sharply demarcated and in the same plane as its surroundings. Histology showed acanthotic epithelium

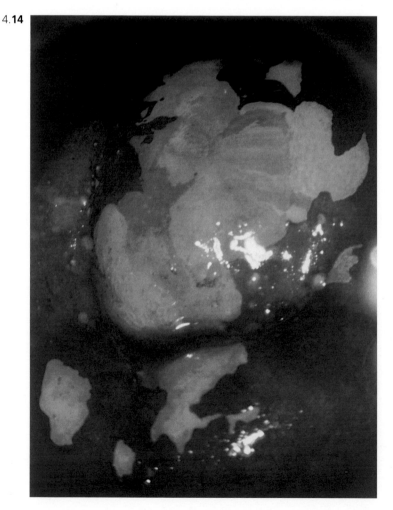

Fig. 4.**14** **Nonsuspicious iodine-yellow area with different color tones,** from yellow to brown, corresponding to sharply demarcated epithelial fields. Histology showed acanthotic epithelium

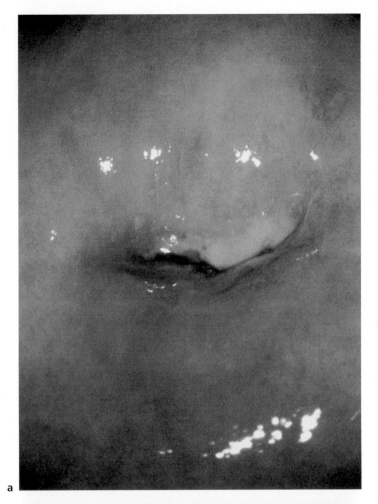

a

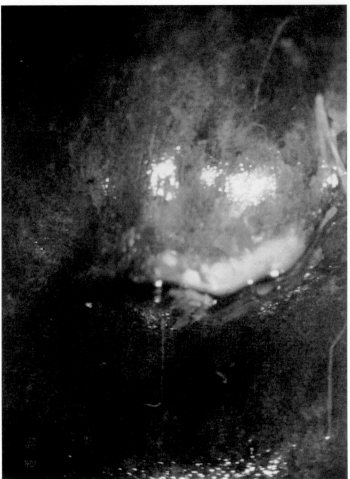

b

Fig. 4.**15a** **Only after the application of acetic acid** does a small, easily missed white area appear on the anterior external os

Fig. 4.**15b** **After application of iodine**, the area on the external os appears bright yellow. Histology showed CIN 2 (H-SIL) in the cervical canal

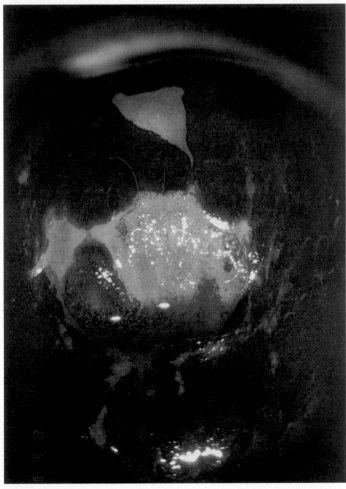

Fig. 4.**16** **Patchy uptake of iodine by a partially atypical transformation zone.** Histology showed carcinoma in situ (CIN 3, H-SIL). On the left, within the transformation zone, there is a small condylomatous area with iodine-positive punctation. At 12 o'clock there is an isolated inconspicuous iodine-yellow area

6. The colposcopist who uses the Schiller test routinely will often see well-demarcated areas with a characteristic canary yellow color that otherwise escape colposcopic detection. Such an area, which is otherwise inconspicuous, is referred to as an *inconspicuous iodine-yellow area,* and is usually due to acanthotic epithelium (Fig. 4.**5**).

If the exact location of the inconspicuous iodine-yellow area has been noted, colposcopic examination after the effect of iodine has subsided can detect a fine color difference between this area and normal squamous epithelium (Fig. 7.**51**).

7. Not only the nuances of color, but also the borders between normal and altered epithelia can be viewed to advantage with the help of iodine. The epithelial borders within colposcopic lesions also become distinct (Fig. 4.**4**; see also Figs. 9.**19b** and 10.**2**). There is no better way to demonstrate the sharpness and clarity of epithelial borders. This is of great diagnostic import, as poorly circumscribed colposcopic areas are hardly ever significant (Figs. 4.**6**–4.**9**, 4.**11**).

Table 4.**1** summarizes the various iodine reactions which are of diagnostic value.

Table 4.**1** Normal and abnormal reactions with iodine

1. Iodine positive = deep brown = normal glycogen-containing epithelium
2. Iodine negative = no reaction with iodine solution = columnar epithelium, immature transformation zone, inflammatory lesions
3. Weak reaction with iodine = various lighter shades of brown = waning estrogen effect, normal transformation zone in its various stages of development
4. Iodine-yellow area = characteristic canary yellow discoloration = mosaic, punctation, atypical transformation zone
5. Colposcopically inconspicuous (nonsuspicous) iodine yellow area
6. Sharp demarcation in cases of (4) and (5)

References

1 Burghardt E. Über die atypische Umwandlungszone. Geburtshilfe Frauenheilkd 1959;19:676.
2 Friedell GH, Hertig AT, Younge PA. The problem of early stromal invasion in carcinoma in situ of the uterine cervix. Arch Pathol 1958;66:494.
3 Hinselmann H. Die Essigsäureprobe: Ein Bestandteil der erweiterten Kolposkopie. Dtsch Med Wochenschr 1938;64:40.
4 Hinselmann H. Die Kolposkopie. Wuppertal: Girardet, 1954.
5 Kern G. Carcinoma in situ. Berlin: Springer, 1964.
6 Schiller W. Jodpinselung und Abschabung des Portioepithels. Zentralbl Gynäkol 1929;53:1056.
7 Schiller W. Early diagnosis of carcinoma of the cervix. Surg Gynecol Obstet 1933;56:210.
8 Schiller W. Early diagnosis of carcinoma of the portio uteri. Am J Surg 1934;26:269.
9 Schiller W. Zur Frühdiagnose des Karzinoms der Portio uteri. Monatsschr Krebsbekämpfung 1934;2:7.
10 Schiller W. Pathology of the cervix. Am J Obstet Gynecol 1937;34:430.
11 Schiller W. Leukoplakia, leukokeratosis, and carcinoma of the cervix. Am J Obstet Gynecol 1938;35:17.
12 Younge PA. A gynecologist's evaluation of methods of early cancer diagnosis. In: Homburger F, Fishman WH, eds. The laboratory diagnosis of cancer of the cervix. New York: Karger, 1956.
13 Younge PA. Cancer of the uterine cervix: a preventable disease. Obstet Gynecol 1957;10:469.
14 Younge PA, Kevorkian AY. Carcinoma in situ of the cervix: the problems of detection and evaluation in regard to the therapy. London: Churchill, 1959. (Ciba foundation study group 3:83–103.)

5

The Colposcopic Examination

Positioning the Patient

The patient is examined in the lithotomy position. We prefer stirrups, which support only the feet and heels and allow bending of the knees and good abduction of the thighs (Fig. 5.**1**). The table should be adjustable to the required height.

Exposure of the Cervix

The self-retaining duckbill speculum (see Fig. 3.**3**) can be used to expose the cervix. When inserted and opened, the speculum is correctly positioned and held by the examiner's free hand (Fig. 5.**2**). The speculum should be as large as the patient can tolerate without discomfort. The tips of the blades should be in the vaginal fornices, which should be widely separated. This procedure provides a good view of the cervix and surrounding vaginal fornices. It also everts the lips of the multiparous cervix, allowing the lower portion of the endocervical canal to come into view; in this way, a pseudoectopy can be produced. The examination is useless if the vagina and cervix are poorly exposed because important lesions can be missed and wrong diagnoses made.

We prefer vaginal retractors with a flat anterior and a grooved posterior blade, available in different lengths and widths (see Fig. 3.**2**). Placing the tips of the retractors in the fornices results in good exposure of the vagina and at times eversion of the lower canal. It is a great advantage to have a wide field of view at the vaginal opening (Fig. 5.**3**). The fact that the anterior retractor must be held in place by an assistant is a drawback (Fig. 5.**1**), but the assistant's free hand can expedite the examination. Even the patient herself can hold the anterior retractor once it is in the right position. The colposcopist guides the posterior blade and conducts the examination at the same time (Fig. 5.**4**).

The retractors are particularly useful if the cervix is difficult to expose because of anatomic deformity, such as stenosis or atrophy. In such circumstances, a second anterior speculum can be inserted laterally on one side (Fig. 5.**5**).

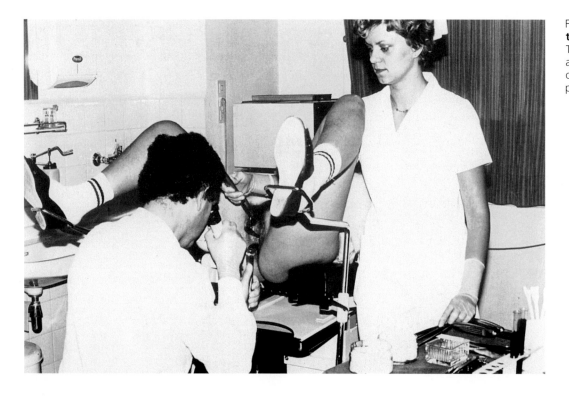

Fig. 5.**1 Colposcopic examination using vaginal retractors.** The anterior retractor is held by an assistant, who can also perform other tasks. Accessories are displayed on the tray

Initial Inspection

After exposing the cervix, one should assess the nature of the cervicovaginal secretions and note any obvious lesion in the fornices or on the cervix.

Removal of Mucus and Discharge

Vaginal secretions, which obscure the view, are removed gently with swabs held by forceps (see Fig. 3.**4** and 3.**5**). Loss of epithelium and bleeding due to traumatic manipulation should be avoided.

First Colposcopic Examination

The cervix and exposed portions of the vagina can now be inspected colposcopically. Differences in color, surface contour, and margins between lesions and normal tissues should be carefully noted.

Special attention should be paid to the blood vessels, which are better displayed at this stage of the examination than after the application of acetic acid (see Fig. 7.**31**). For this purpose, the green filter is particularly useful, as it shows the terminal angioarchitecture etched out in black, allowing a degree of discrimination not otherwise achieved. We recommend routine use of this filter.

Acetic Acid Test

The whole cervix, and particularly all visible lesions, are carefully dabbed with swabs saturated with 3% acetic acid (see Fig. 3.**5**). The swabs are held with forceps, which also squeezes out excess fluid. The lesions should be swabbed, not wiped, to avoid injury to the epithelium. Excess acetic acid can be soaked up by dry swabs.

Second Colposcopic Examination

The most important part of the colposcopic examination follows the application of acetic acid. The well-displayed changes can now be subjected to detailed scrutiny, which allows their definition and assessment. It is particularly important to observe any color change and swelling of the epithelium caused by the acetic acid. These are two important criteria by which colposcopic findings can be classified (see Chapter 9). It is important to realize that it may take a minute or so for maximal changes to develop.

Schiller (Iodine) Test

Approximately 3 ml of 1% Lugol's iodine is poured into the posterior fornix (Fig. 5.**6**) from a test tube (see Fig. 3.**5**). By manipulating the anterior retractor, the cervix is immersed in the fluid pool. Alternatively, one can apply the iodine with swabs. Again, any excess is removed with dry swabs.

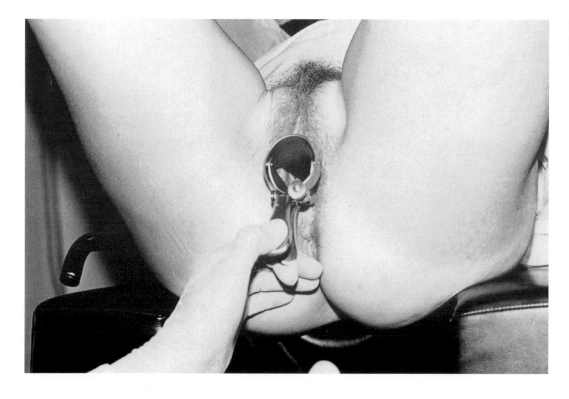

Fig. 5.**2 Examination with the duckbill speculum,** which is easily manipulated by one hand

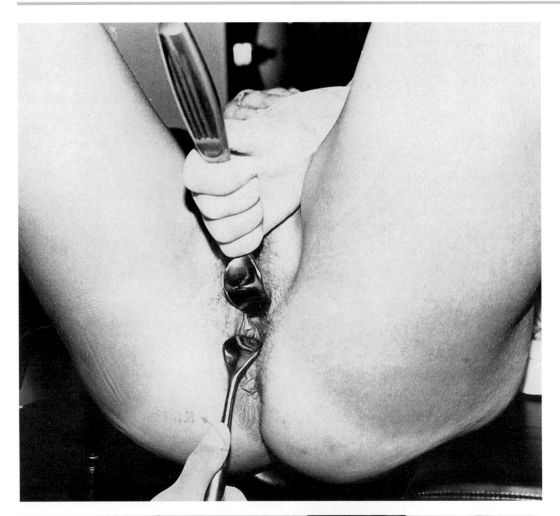

Fig. 5.**3** **Appropriately sized retractors allow optimal exposure.** The anterior retractor is held by an assistant

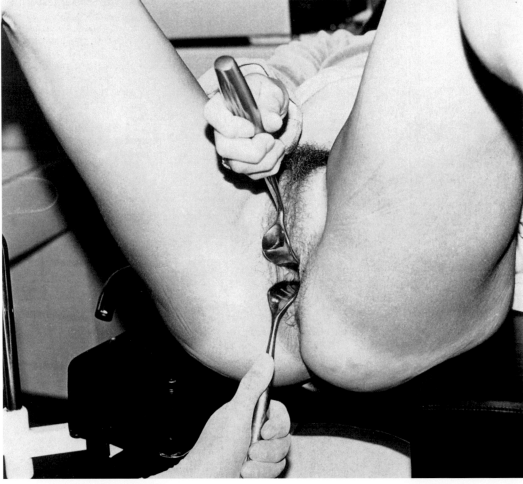

Fig. 5.**4** **If an assistant is not available, the anterior retractor can be held by the patient** once it has been properly positioned by the examiner

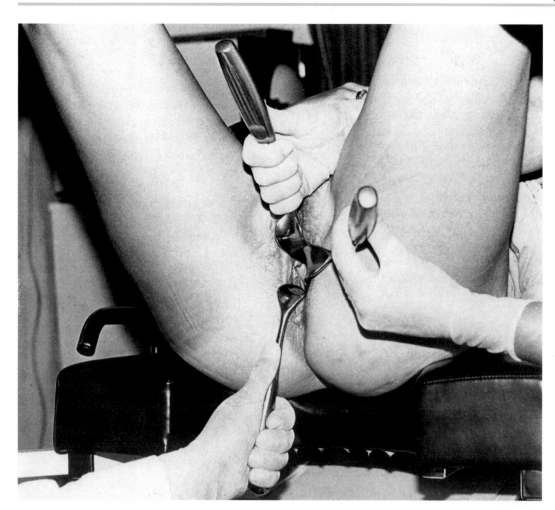

Fig. 5.**5**   Exposure can be increased by inserting a third retractor

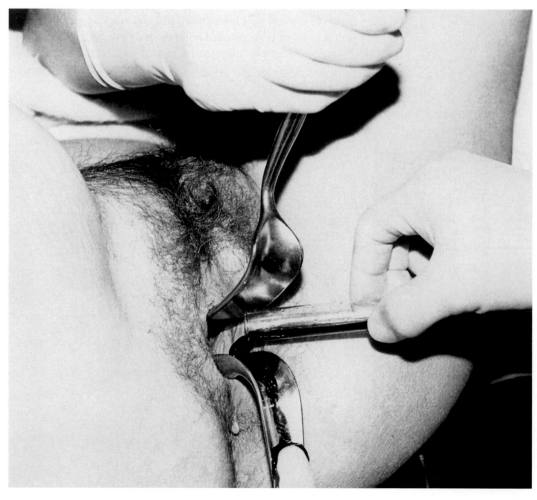

Fig. 5.**6**   **The Schiller test** is performed by pouring several milliliters of Lugol's iodine into the posterior fornix. The cervix is then immersed in the pool by manipulating the anterior retractor. Excess fluid is removed with dry swabs. This method produces more uniform staining than using wet swabs

Final Colposcopic Inspection

The final step in the examination, which follows the application of iodine, was introduced by Hinselmann soon after the publication of Schiller's test, but is nowadays omitted by many colposcopists. The experienced colposcopist, however, would not do without it (see Chapters 4 and 9). First, iodine can reveal typically yellow, sharply demarcated lesions previously unsuspected. Second, the exact color tone a lesion assumes may be of diagnostic value (see p. 23). Finally, there is no better way of demonstrating the sharp borders between normal and newly formed epithelia than with Lugol's iodine. Evaluation of a seemingly typical transformation zone is not complete without the Schiller test.

Following the examination of the cervix, the retractors are withdrawn slowly, so that any changes in the vagina may be seen.

Documentation of the Colposcopic Findings

This is carried out with photographs or sketches. To avoid taking too many pictures, it is best to photograph the cervix after the application of acetic acid. For further details, see Chapter 11.

Obtaining Smears for Exfoliative Cytology

Optimal samples for cervical cytology require that they be taken from the proper location (the area where cervical carcinomas are most likely to arise) with an appropriate instrument.

The cervix and vagina are exposed with retractors so that the smear can be obtained under direct vision. The smear should be taken at the beginning of the examination, before applying acetic acid for colposcopy. Vaginal douches and local medications should not have been used within the preceding few days. The surface of the cervix should not be wiped.

Most cervical carcinomas and their precursors develop in the transformation zone between the squamous epithelium and columnar epithelium. The transformation zone is usually near the external os of the cervix and moves upward into the cervical canal with age.

A variety of instruments to obtain samples have been developed in different sizes and shapes (Fig. 5.7). For routine cytology smears can be obtained with a wet cotton-tipped swab and smeared onto a slide. An Ayre's spatula, which has a concavity at one end, can also be used. Small brushes are better than spatulas for obtaining material from the cervical canal.

Smears can also be taken under colposcopic guidance. Attention can be directed towards colposcopic abnormalities, but the entire cervix should be sampled.

Target Biopsy

Biopsies should be taken only after the colposcopic examination has been completed. Depending on the site of the suspicious lesion, either a punch biopsy or endocervical curettage should be carried out. Occasionally, both procedures are necessary.

Fig. 5.**7** Instruments for obtaining samples for cervical cytology
a Ayre's spatula **b** Cotton-tipped swab **c** Cytobrush **d** Cervix brush **e** Expanding brush **f–j** Szalay spatulas

Punch Biopsy

The instrument for punch biopsy is pistol-shaped, with a long shaft (see Fig. 3.**6**). Under colposcopic control, the instrument is guided to the area where the biopsy specimen is to be obtained. Although the cervix tends to slip away on pressure, it is usually easy to grasp and remove the desired tissue with the biopsy forceps. The procedure is virtually painless. The specimen is approximately 3 mm in size, and is covered on one side by epithelium. Several specimens may be taken from larger lesions. Bleeding is usually mild, but may occasionally be heavy. The patient should be given some type of sanitary pad. We prefer a sterile tampon (see Fig. 3.**5**), which is shown to the patient prior to insertion and which she is instructed to remove on the same day. Bleeding always stops within a few hours.

If the cervix gives way under pressure or slips away from the instrument, it must be "fixed." This is best done with a single-toothed tenaculum (see Fig. 3.**7**). The point at which the cervix is grasped must be away from any lesions. This manipulation is not painful.

The tissue remains in the concavity of the instrument's jaw. The instrument is then immersed in fixative in a specimen jar, and the specimen is shaken free.

Loop Diathermy Excision

A variety of wire loops have been used in Europe for decades for diathermy excision or cervical biopsies. Cartier (1977) has revived and perfected the technique. The procedure can be performed under local anesthesia by injecting a solution of ornipressin. It is appropriate for lesions of different sizes that can be removed with a margin of healthy tissue. The excision is performed with a very small amount of pressure on the loop. After removal of the tissue, the wound, which hardly bleeds after infiltration, is coagulated with a ball electrode.

Endocervical Curettage

First, the patient must be warned that this procedure may be uncomfortable, as it is done without a general anesthetic. Fixing the cervix, as described for punch biopsy, is rarely necessary.

The procedure is performed with sharp, spoon-shaped or grooved curettes (see Fig. 3.**6**); the latter are particularly useful for insertion through a narrow os. The canal is scraped in a circumferential manner. Tissue that remains in the cavity of the jaws of the instrument may be rinsed in the fixative. Residual tissue fragments on the surface of the cervix or around the os can be removed with forceps and then placed in fixative.

During the curettage, the consistency of the cervical wall should be noted. If it is firm and regular, it is unlikely to harbor a deeply invasive carcinoma; such tissue is friable and would disintegrate during curettage. Bleeding is not usually excessive. Nevertheless, the patient is given a sanitary pad or a tampon.

Chrobak's Sound

The uterine sound test devised by the Viennese gynecologist Chrobak (1840–1910) is a simple way to distinguish between benign and malignant tissue. It is particularly useful in assessing purely endophytic or only slightly ulcerating carcinomas and to distinguish between benign papillomas and exophytic carcinomas. The sound (see Fig. 3.**8**) easily penetrates cancerous tissue on light pressure, as if going into butter. According to the depth of penetration, even the volume of the tumor can be estimated. Conversely, the sound encounters elastic resistance when in contact with normal tissues or benign tumors. The sound can traumatize atypical epithelium but not normal epithelium.

Duration of Colposcopic Examination

Careful performance of all steps should not take longer than 3 minutes. Another 2 to 3 minutes may be added if a biopsy is to be taken. It must be stressed again that the best result is achieved by the routine use of colposcopy. Once the colposcopist has learned how to handle the instruments and how to interpret cervical changes, 3 minutes' time should be ample.

Reference

Cartier R. Practical colposcopy. Basel: S. Karger, 1977.

6
Colposcopic Terminology

Hinselmann's Nomenclature

At first, Hinselmann (6) recognized only a few colposcopic findings, which he divided into *normal* and *pathologic:*

1. *Normal findings*
   Original mucosa
   Ectopy
   Transformation zone
2. *Pathologic findings*
   Portio leukoplakia
   Ground of leukoplakia (punctation)
   "Felderung" (mosaic)

When Hinselmann removed the keratin layer from the surfaces of leukoplakia he detected on their "ground" a punctation. He also found *"Felderung"* to be associated with leukoplakia.

Hinselmann (4, 5) referred to the pathologic findings, which he believed were always due to epithelial precursors of cervical carcinoma, collectively as the *matrix area.* Only later (7) did he acknowledge the existence of an atypical transformation zone as originally described by Treite (10).

Hinselmann also recognized the significance of *true erosion* (6), which he distinguished from what was previously known simply as *erosion* and is now referred to, in contrast to leukoplakia, as *erythroplakia.* He also suggested that erosions appeared in areas previously occupied by atypical epithelium, which he found to be fragile and of low cohesiveness. The quite flat ulcer caused by endophytic carcinoma was also included in this schema.

Table 6.**1** **Colposcopic terminology** (Rome 1990)

I **Normal colposcopic findings**
A Original squamous epithelium
B Columnar epithelium
C Normal transformation zone
II **Abnormal colposcopic findings**
A Within the transformation zone
1 Acetowhite epithelium*
a Flat
b Micropapillary or microconvoluted
2 Punctation*
3 Mosaic*
4 Leukoplakia*
5 Iodine-negative area
6 Atypical vessels
B Outside the transformation zone, e.g., ectocervix, vagina
1 Acetowhite epithelium*
a Flat
b Micropapillary or microconvoluted
2 Punctation*
3 Mosaic*
4 Leukoplakia*
5 Iodine-negative area
6 Atypical vessels
III **Colposcopically suspect invasive carcinoma**
IV **Unsatisfactory colposcopy**
A Squamocolumnar junction not visible
B Severe inflammation or severe atrophy
C Cervix not visible
V **Miscellaneous findings**
A Non acetowhite micropapillary surface
B Exophytic condyloma
C Inflammation
D Atrophy
E Ulcer
F Other

* Indicates minor or major change

Minor changes
    Acetowhite epithelium
    Fine mosaic
    Fine punctation
    Thin leukoplakia

Major changes
    Dense acetowhite epithelium
    Coarse mosaic
    Coarse punctation
    Thick leukoplakia
    Atypical vessels
    Erosion

Wespi's Nomenclature

Wespi (11) divided colposcopic findings into four groups; normal established carcinoma, atypical epithelium, and findings of uncertain significance:

1. *Normal appearance of the portio*
   Original portio mucosa
   Ectopy
   Transformation zone
2. *Established portio carcinoma*
3. *Atypical portio epithelium*
   Leukoplakia
   "Ground" (punctation)
   "Felderung" (mosaic)
   Colposcopically inconspicuous iodine-negative area
4. *Findings of uncertain significance*

This nomenclature distinguished for the first time between ground (punctation) and *Felderung* (mosaic) on the one hand, and leukoplakia on the other. The concept of a colposcopically inconspicuous iodine-negative area was also new. Prominent among the findings of uncertain significance was a *red area* mainly corresponding to *true erosion.*

The International Terminology

A new colposcopic terminology was presented at the World Congress for Colposcopy and Cervical Pathology in Rome in 1990 (9).

This terminology is an improvement insofar as it takes into account the fact that identical colposcopic lesions can be found both within and outside the transformation zone. Also, the sudivision of mosaic lesions and leukoplakia into minor changes and major changes (albeit in footnotes) implies a certain qualitative assessment.

The terminology used in this book is shown in Table 6.**2**. It generally corresponds to the international terminology updated in Barcelona 2002 (see Table 1, p. 3), but clarifies its weaknesses (12).

Table 6.**2** **Terminology used in this book**

I	Normal colposcopic findings
	A Original squamous epithelium
	B Ectopy (columnar epithelium)
	C Transformation zone
II	Doubtful colposcopic findings
	A Thin leukoplakia
	B Fine punctation
	C Fine mosaic
	D White epithelium (atypical transformation zone)
	E Colposcopically inconspicuous (nonsuspicious) iodine-yellow area
III	Suspicious colposcopic findings
	A Coarse leukoplakia
	B Coarse punctation
	C Coarse mosaic
	D White epithelium (atypical transformation zone)
	E Erosion (ulcer)
	F Suspicious invasive carcinoma
IV	Invasive carcinoma
V	Miscellaneous findings
	A Condylomas
	B Polyps
	C Inflammatory changes
	D Atrophic changes
	E Others

References

1 Almendral AC, Seidl S. Colposcopical terminology. Chairmen's report. In: Burghardt E, Holzer E, Jordan JA; eds. Cervical pathology and colposcopy. Stuttgart: Thieme, 1978:134–135.

2 Burghardt E, Coupez F, Dexeus S, et al. A European proposal for a classification of colposcopic findings. Cervix 1989;7:251–4.

3 Cartier R. Practical Colposcopy. Basel: Karger, 1977.

4 Hinselmann H. Ausgewählte Gesichtspunkte zur Beurteilung des Zusammenhanges der "Matrixbezirke" und des Karzinoms der sichtbaren Abschnitte des weiblichen Genitaltraktes. Z Geburtshilfe 1933;104:228.

5 Hinselmann H. Die klinische und mikroskopische Frühdiagnose des Portiokarzinoms. Arch Gynäkol 1934;156:239.

6 Hinselmann H. Die Kolposkopie. Wuppertal: Girardet, 1954.

7 Hinselmann H. Kolposkopische Studien, vol 1. Leipzig: VEB Thieme, 1954.

8 Stafl A. New nomenclature for colposcopy. Obstet Gynecol 1976;48:123.

9 Stafl A, Wilbanks G. An international terminology of colposcopy. Report of the Nomenclature Committee of the International Federation of Cervical Pathology and Colposcopy. Obstet Gynecol 1991; 77:313.

10 Treite P. Die Frühdiagnose des Plattenepithel-Karzinoms am Collum uteri. Stuttgart: Enke, 1944.

11 Wespi H. Early carcinoma of the uterine cervix: pathogenesis and detection. New York: Grune and Stratton, 1949.

12 Walker P, Dexeus S, De Palo G, Barrasso R, Campion M, Girardi F, Jakob C, Roy M. International terminology of colposcopy: an updated report from the International Federation for Cervical Pathology and Colposcopy Obstet Gynecol 101:175–177, 2003

7

Colposcopic Morphology

Introduction

The best way to describe and depict colposcopic findings is with colpophotographs. The illustrations here have been chosen to portray as faithfully as possible all the important changes encountered in daily practice. Colposcopy can be understood only if it is appreciated that the same colposcopic appearance can be produced by a number of biologically different processes. This apparent diagnostic paradox can be resolved only with a knowledge of the underlying histologies. The colposcopic literature neglects the fact that a lesion is often a composite of a number of quite different epithelial types of differing significance, though sharing a common origin. This is attested to by the constant location of the various epithelia and their clear demarcation from each other. These features are the key for the understanding of colposcopic diagnosis and parameters without which no concept of the morphogenesis of cervical carcinoma can be formulated. The relationship between cervical pathology and colposcopic diagnosis is fundamental and reciprocal.

Normal Colposcopic Appearances

Original Squamous Epithelium

Like any normal surface squamous epithelium, the native, original squamous epithelium is smooth and uninterrupted by gland openings (Fig. 7.1). This sets it apart from normal squamous epithelium that has arisen through metaplasia. More detailed observation of a surface covered by the latter type of epithelium reveals the presence of gland openings and retention cysts, which indicate that the area was originally occupied by columnar epithelium (see Fig. 7.1). The original squamous epithelium during the reproductive period displays a reddish color that can vary from pale to intense pink during the various phases of the menstrual cycle. The deep-brown stain with iodine reflects its glycogen content (see Fig. 4.8b).

Fig. 7.**1** **Original squamous epithelium** of the reproductive period. The surface is completely smooth and displays a fresh reddish color

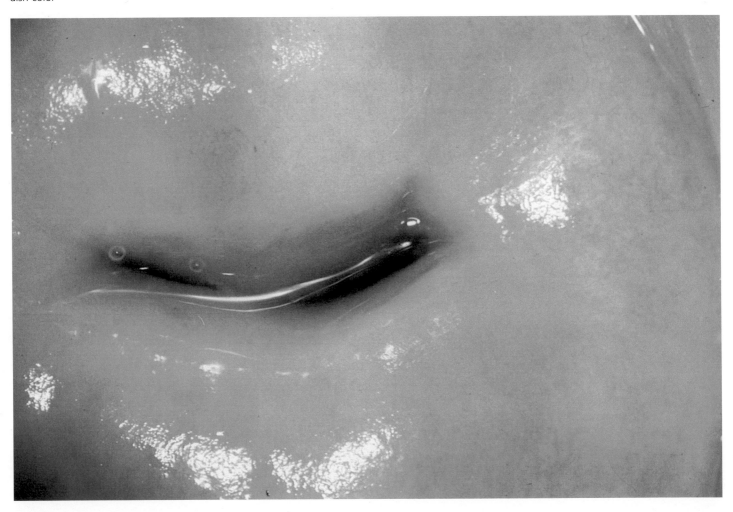

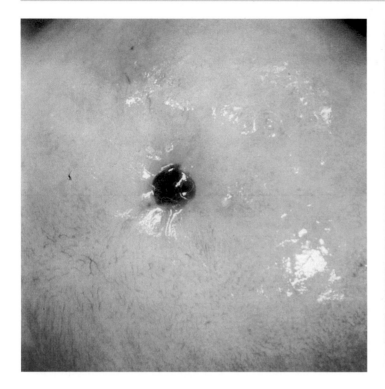

Fig. 7.**2a** **Atrophic squamous epithelium in a postmenopausal patient.** Fine blood vessels shine through the thin epithelium, which appears pale pink to yellowish

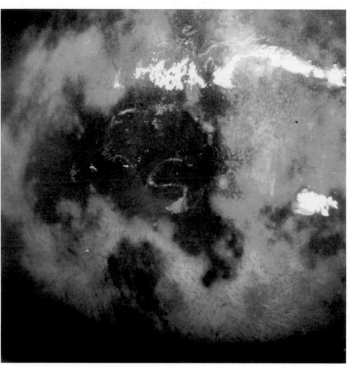

Fig. 7.**2b** The same cervix after application of iodine. The characteristic stippled appearance is due to focal glycogen retention

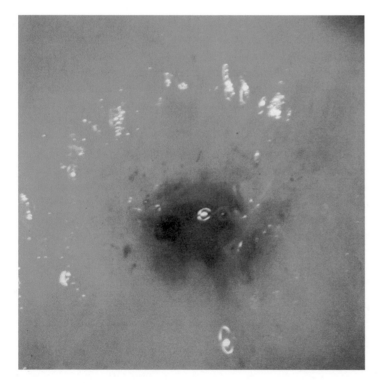

Fig. 7.**3** The loss of glycogen is uniform in the atrophic epithelium of an elderly patient, resulting in homogeneous yellow staining with iodine

Atrophic Squamous Epithelium

After menopause, in the absence of estrogen replacement, the squamous epithelium becomes thin and devoid of glycogen and the stromal blood supply diminishes. These changes result in a pale epithelium that can show a fine network of capillaries (Fig. 7.**2a**).

The epithelial thinning and loss of glycogen are patchy. This results in a stippled appearance with iodine because of its irregular uptake (Fig. 7.**2b**). In the elderly, the epithelium assumes a uniform light brown to yellow discoloration as a result of complete loss of glycogen (Fig. 7.**3**).

The thin epithelial covering is fragile and makes the terminal vessels vulnerable to minor trauma, which can result in erosions and subepithelial hemorrhages (Fig. 7.**4**).

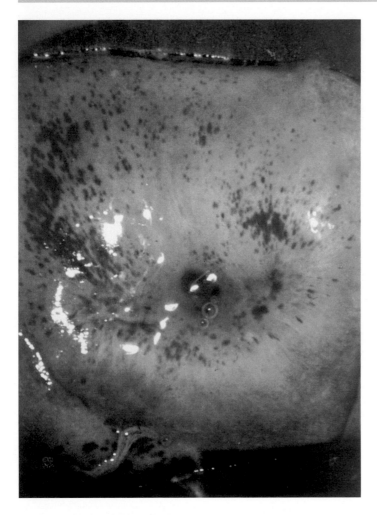

Fig. 7.**4** With advancing age, the squamous epithelium becomes fragile. Subepithelial hemorrhages may appear during vaginal examination. Note the fine vessels that stream toward the os

Ectopy (Columnar Epithelium)

Ideally the original squamocolumnar junction is situated at the external os. According to the size, shape and patulousnous of the external os, varying portions of the canal may be visible. In patulous cervices, the architecture of endocervical mucosa can be seen clearly (Fig. 7.**5**).

In some circumstances, the columnar epithelium is situated on the ectocervix at some distance from the external os. This is referred to as *ectopy*. The alternative term *columnar epithelium* is quite acceptable, but does not indicate its ectopic location. In cases of marked eversion of the endocervical mucosa, its rugose architecture becomes evident (Fig. 7.**6**). In such cases, it may be more accurate to speak of an *ectropion* rather than ectopy.

Ectopy is more often apparent than real. The separated blades of the speculum spread out the fornices and evert the endocervical canal, so that it appears as part of the covering of the ectocervix (Fig. 7.**7**).

True ectopy appears classically as a "red patch" (Fig. 7.**8a**). Macroscopically it may look highly suspicious to the inexperienced examiner. More detailed colposcopic examination reveals its unique papillary architecture, which identifies its real nature. It is always iodine-negative (Fig. 7.**8b**).

Ectopy is usually covered by mucus secreted by the columnar epithelium. Acetic acid helps to remove the mucus (see p. 33), revealing a distinctive papillary structure. At the same time, it causes the tissue to swell, throwing the mucosal architecture into sharp relief, and giving the papillae a grape-like appearance. The intense red of the red patch changes to pink or whitish (Figs. 7.**9**, 7.**10**).

The *squamocolumnar junction* is usually sharp and step-like (Figs. 7.**5**, 7.**10** and 7.**11**). Careful observation of the margin, however, often reveals a slender seam, the white color and gland openings of which indicate the initiation of transformation (Figs. 7.**7** and 7.**9**). It is important to pay close attention to the margins in ectopy so as not to overlook significant colposcopic lesions.

Ectopic columnar epithelium is less resilient and more vulnerable to trauma than squamous epithelium. It is subject to contact bleeding even during hasty speculum examination. Any contact bleeding, however, should raise the possibility of a carcinoma. Although neoplastic papillary fronds tend to be coarse and irregular, they can be mistaken for benign changes.

Fig. 7.**5** **The original squamo-columnar junction** of this gaping cervix is most distinct. The anterior lip displays a thin rim of transformation zone. The rugose structure of the endocervical mucosa is clearly seen

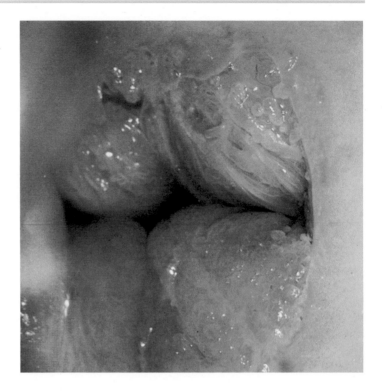

Fig. 7.**6** **Eversion of the endocervical mucosa,** with its rugose architecture thrown into sharp relief. This can be referred to as *ectropion*

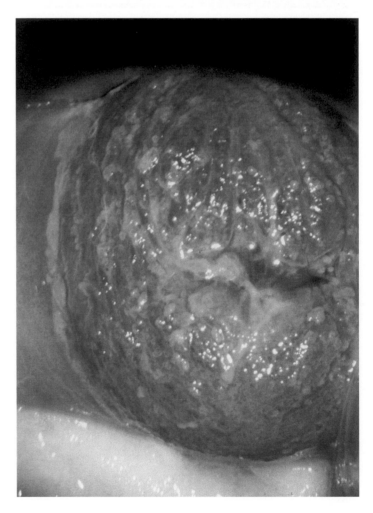

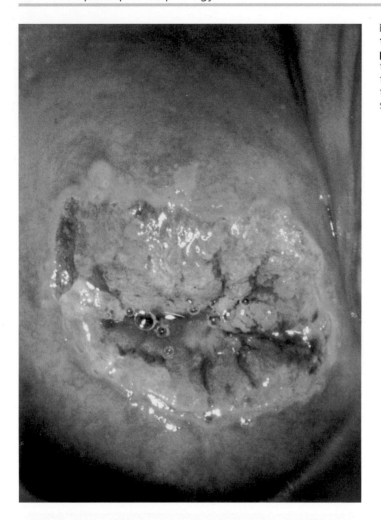

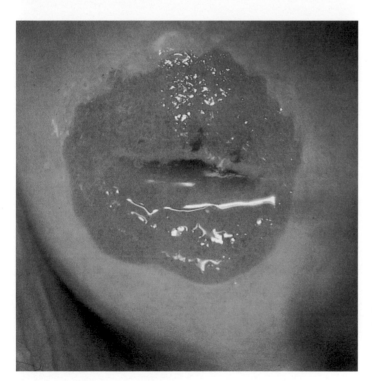

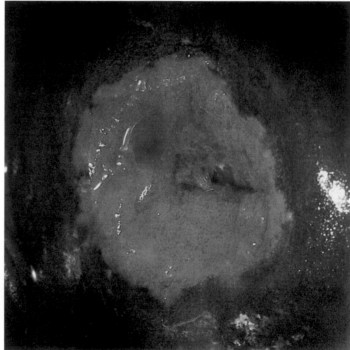

Fig. 7.**7   Apparent eversion (ectopy) of a cervix with a patulous os,** due to wide separation of the speculum. A thin rim of transformation zone is visible near the junction with the original squamous epithelium

Fig. 7.**8 a   Ectopy before application of acetic acid.** The gland openings at the 10-o'clock position indicate preceding transformation

Fig. 7.**8 b   An ectopy does not stain with iodine;** it is merely discolored by the thin film covering it. The demarcation from the deep-brown original squamous epithelium is indistinct

a
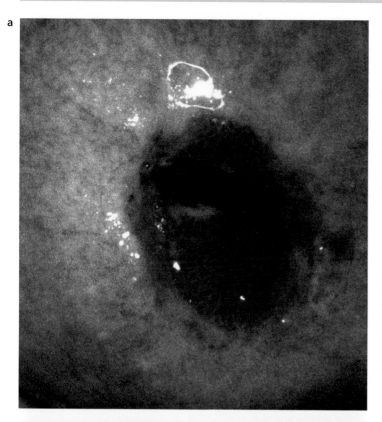

b
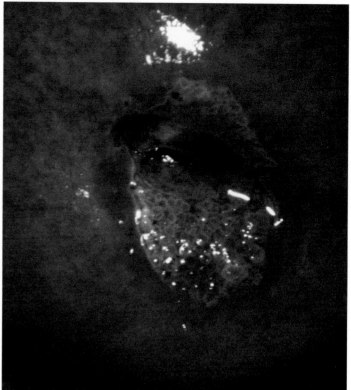

c
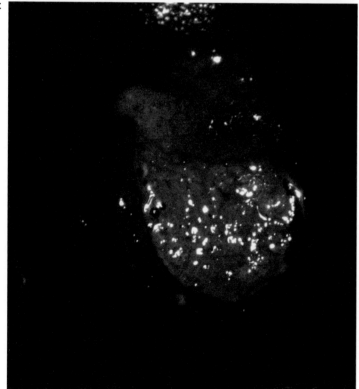

Fig. 7.**9**   Small red area on the anterior and posterior lip of the external os

a Before application of acetic acid **b** After application of 3% acetic acid **c** After application of iodine. The columnar epithelium does not stain. The transformation zone at the margins is identifiable by the incomplete staining of the new squamous cell epithelium

Fig. 7.**10** **Classical appearance of ectopy after application of acetic acid.** The grape-like structure is unmistakable. Note the whitish rim of transformation zone at the periphery ▷

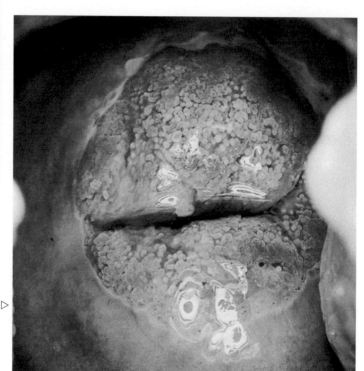

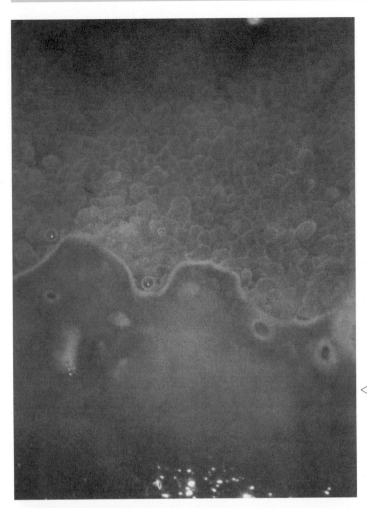

Transformation Zone

The transformation zone can appear as a nonspecific red area. Sometimes there is a fine vascular pattern (Fig. 7.**12a**). Application of acetic acid turns the previously red epithelium grayish-white. Within the transformation zone, there are openings of cervical glands and small islands of residual columnar epithelium. The demarcation from the original squamous epithelium is indistinct (Fig. 7.**12b**).

◁ Fig. 7.**11** **Step-like border between the grape-like structure of the ectopy and the squamous epithelium.** Note the gland openings at the periphery of the squamous epithelium, indicating completed transformation at the edge of the previously larger ectopic area

Fig. 7.**12a** **Typical transformation zone** before the application of acetic acid. There are small, unremarkable vessels at the edge of the reddish area on the posterior lip of the cervix

Fig. 7.**12b** After application of acetic acid the previously reddish epithelium is grayish-white. Gland openings and small islands of residual columnar epithelium are signs of the transformation zone

7.**12a**

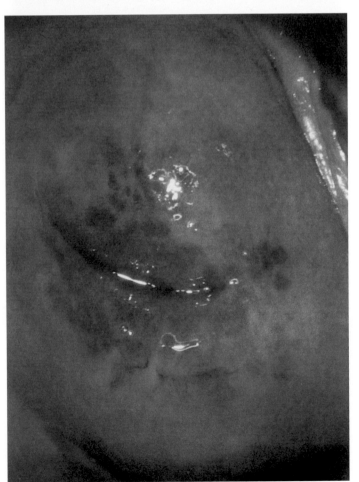

7.**12b**

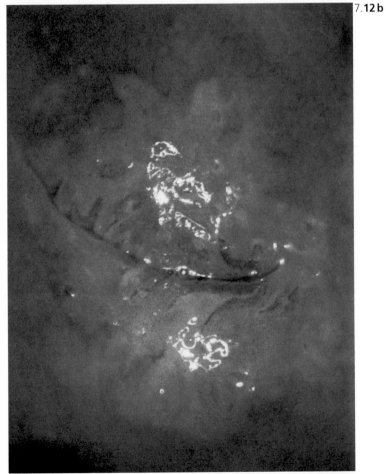

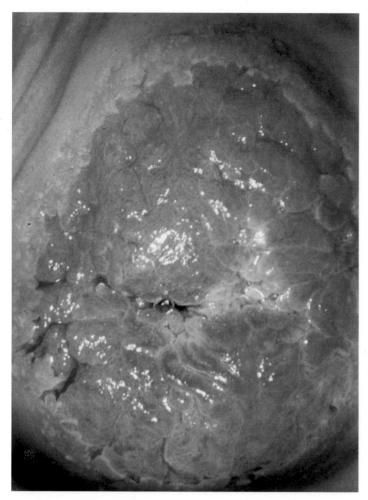

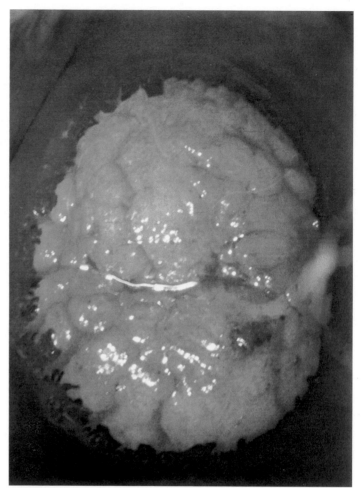

Fig. 7.**13 a** **Transformation zone.** Centrally, within this ectopic area, the villi become plumper and fuse to form a flat surface eventually

Fig. 7.**13 b** The same case following application of iodine. The transformed epithelium is already mature and contains glycogen. Gland openings are well displayed. The central part does not take up iodine, which merely covers it like a veil

The process of transformation characteristically begins at the squamocolumnar junction. The flat epithelial seam around the periphery of an ectopy can be distinguished from the original squamous as well as columnar epithelium by its variable color and by the presence of gland openings (Figs. 4.**2**, 7.**11**, 7.**13**). It is impossible to tell colposcopically whether the transformation process at this site is due to ascending healing or squamous metaplasia.

Pari passu with peripheral transformation of an ectopy, the surface contour of its central portion undergoes changes. The papillae become coarse and fused, resulting in only slight fissuring of the surface. These changes signify the initiation of squamous metaplasia. Fields of metaplastic epithelium within a transformation zone may vary widely in their maturation, easily verifiable by the Schiller test, which is a sensitive indicator of epithelial maturity (Fig. 7.**13 b**).

The topographic progress of the transformation may be haphazard, and its stage of evolution can vary significantly from one part of the periphery to another. Islands of squamous epithelium can appear in a sea of columnar epithelium; these must have arisen by metaplasia (Fig. 7.**14**). The metaplastic epithelium can form tongues or finger-like processes that inter-digitate with intact columnar epithelium (Fig. 7.**15**). Even when most of an ectopy is fully transformed, small islands of columnar epithelium can remain; this appearance is referred to as transformation zone with ectopic rests (Fig. 7.**16**). The study of the same transformation zone over many years is particularly informative.

The transformation of an ectopy may not always proceed to completion. Areas of the newly formed squamous epithelium can fully mature, whereas other parts of an ectopy can remain intact for long periods (Fig. 7.**17**). A fully transformed ectopy (fully developed transformation zone) can closely resemble the "ideal" cervix. The new squamocolumnar junction is situated again at the external os. The squamous epithelium of such a transformation zone can be distinguished from original squamous epithelium only by the presence of gland openings, more prominent vessels (Fig. 7.**18**), or retention cysts (Fig. 7.**19**). Undulations due to numerous retention cysts (nabothian follicles), with long vessels coursing over their surface, are also characteristic (Fig. 7.**20**). The vasculature in such cases is so typical that the presence of deep-seated and otherwise invisible cysts can be easily deduced (see Fig. 9.**10**).

7.**14**

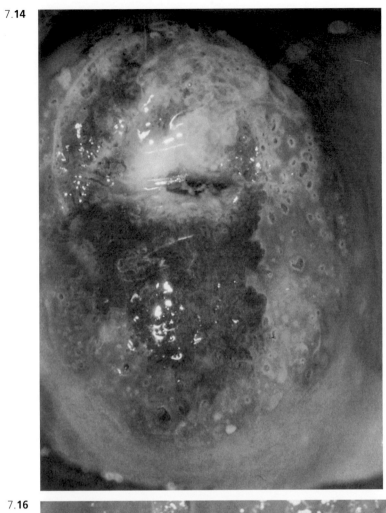

7.**15**

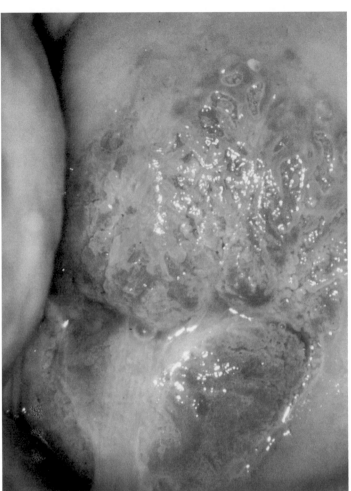

7.**16**

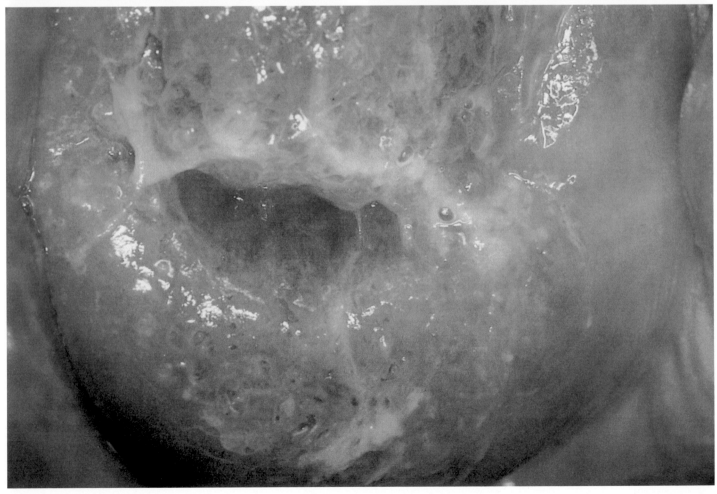

◁ Fig. 7.**14** **Advanced transformation zone.** Here too, the process begins peripherally and spreads toward the center in an irregular manner. Note the smooth surface in spite of the incomplete transformation. There are numerous gland openings

◁ Fig. 7.**15** **Finger-like processes of metaplastic epithelium** extend centrally from the periphery and interdigitate with islands of columnar epithelium. The transformation involves only the anterior lip

◁ Fig. 7.**16** **Transformation zone** with residual islands of grape-like columnar epithelium on the anterior lip

Fig. 7.**17** **Partial transformation.** The transformation zone on the anterior lip takes up only a small portion of the ectopy, which is largely unchanged, apart from enlargement and fusion of its papillae ▷

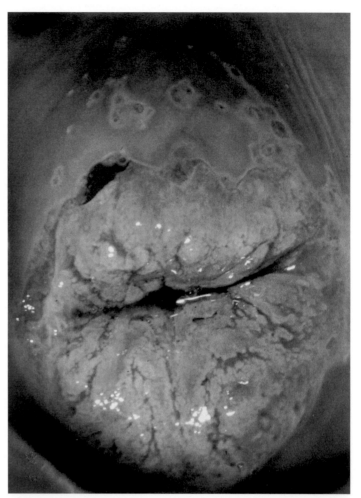

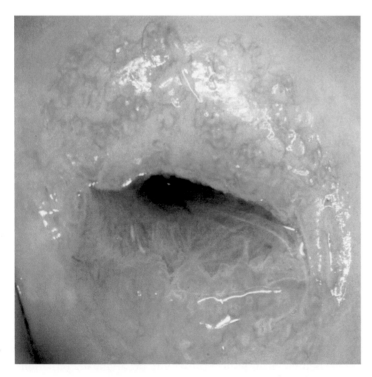

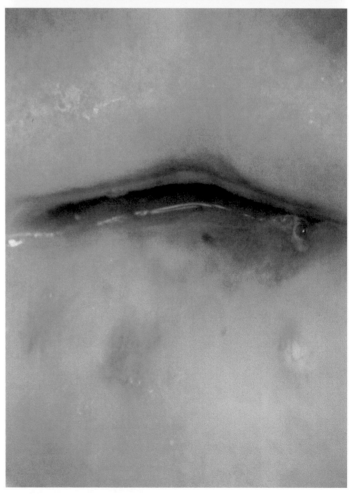

Fig. 7.**18** **Well-established transformation zone.** Although the color of the new squamous epithelium is hardly distinguishable from that of the original, the border of the transformation is marked by fine blood vessels. The new squamocolumnar junction is abrupt

Fig. 7.**19** **Several nabothian follicles covered by smooth squamous epithelium.** They are the only indicators of preceding transformation. Blood vessels characteristically run over the surface of the retention cyst on the right ▷

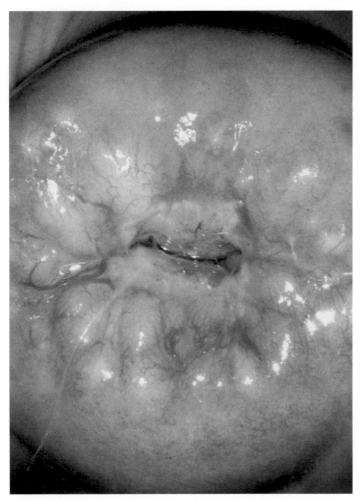

Fig. 7.**20** **Numerous nabothian follicles in an established transformation zone.** The long regularly branching blood vessels that shine through the attenuated epithelium are typical

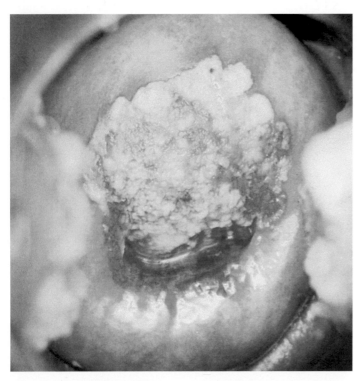

Fig. 7.**21** **Coarse plaque of keratosis** with a partly fissured surface: histologically carcinoma in situ (CIN 3, H-SIL)

Abnormal Colposcopic Findings

Leukoplakia

Leukoplakia can usually be seen with the naked eye (Fig. 7.**21**), but sometimes the colposcope is necessary (Fig. 7.**22**). Histologically leukoplakia corresponds to parakeratosis or true keratinization, which cannot be distinguished colposcopically. A colposcopically delicate white patch, however, usually corresponds to parakeratosis, while hyperkeratosis usually produces a thick, rough-surfaced plaque. Fine leukoplakias are well circumscribed (Fig. 7.**22**), their surface either flat or finely pitted. When keratinization is marked, the margins become obscured by the overlapping horny layer. The surface may be smooth, but is more commonly pitted, and may even have a mosaic appearance. Partial shedding or removal of the keratin can result in a plaque-like appearance, referred to as *plaque-like or thick leukoplakia.*

If the keratin layer is completely removed, the underlying epithelium can display a pattern, often punctation (Fig. 7.**23**) and which Hinselmann designated as the *ground* (base) of leukoplakia (5, 6). Leukoplakia can be found within or outside the transformation zone, in the latter case arising from original squamous epithelium. It is important to appreciate that the type of epithelium underlying leukoplakia cannot be predicted colposcopically. The epithelium may be acanthotic, especially when the leukoplakia is fine. When cornification is more pronounced, the underlying epithelium may show the features of carcinoma in situ (CIN 3, H-SIL), early stromal invasion, and even deeper invasion, or only acanthosis (Figs. 7.**24** and 7.**25**). Even the Schiller test cannot provide further diagnostic clues (Fig. 7.**24b**). Moderate-sized leukoplakias typically stain canary yellow with iodine, which also enhances their sharp demarcation.

Topographic studies have shown that leukoplakia requiring treatment is found only outside the transformation zone and that it corresponds histologically to benign acanthotic epithelium in 62% and to CIN in 38% of cases, respectively (3).

Punctation

As already mentioned, punctation can occur under the keratin layer of a leukoplakia. Usually the punctation is imprinted on a uniform surface which is undisturbed either by gland openings or nabothian follicles or by any other signs of a transformation zone. The degree to which punctation is expressed depends on the type of underlying epithelial abnormality. The type of punctation, as well as of mosaic, is of decisive value in colposcopic evaluation. As stated above, the colposcopist should be aware that similar colposcopic appearances can be due to either benign acanthotic epithelium or atypical epithelium, which differ only in arrangement and degree of expression.

In practice there are two types of punctation of diagnostic importance:

a) *fine punctation* and
b) *coarse punctation.*

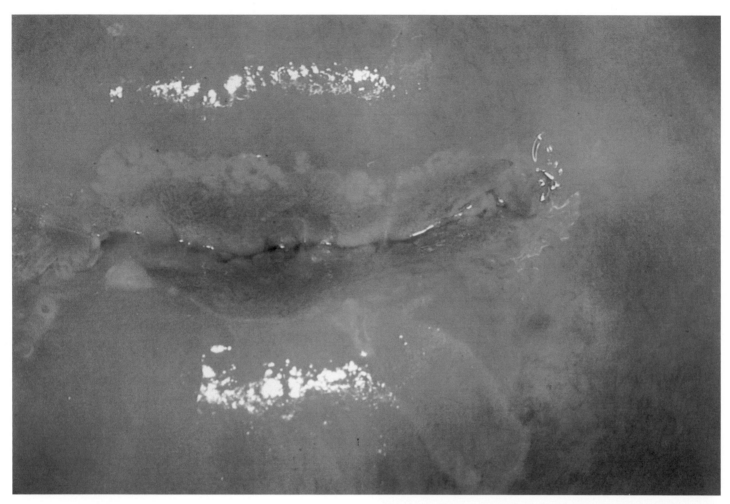

Fig. 7.**22** **Sharply demarcated but only slightly keratotic area** on the posterior lip. Histology showed acanthotic epithelium with parakeratosis. Note the thin seam of transformation zone on the anterior lip

Fig. 7.**23** **Ground of leukoplakia.** Where the keratin layer has been peeled off, punctation appears. Histology showed keratinizing acanthotic epithelium ▷

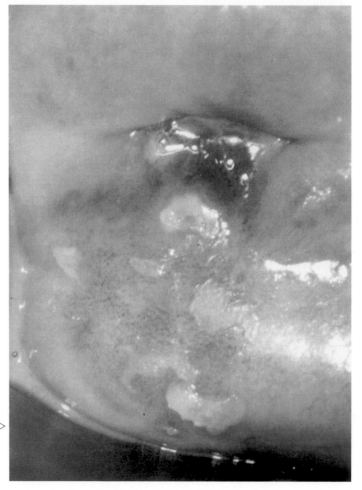

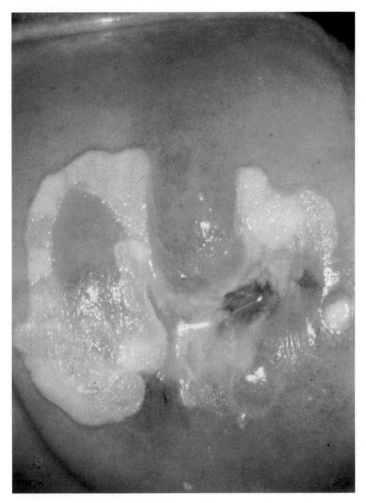

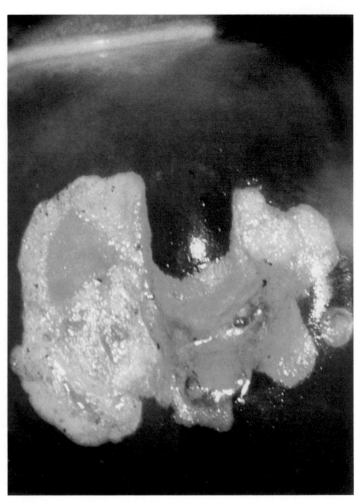

Fig. 7.**24 a** **Pronounced leuko-plakia** displayed by most of a well-circumscribed lesion. Note the sharp border close to the external os at 11-o'clock. Conization showed carcinoma in situ (CIN 3, H-SIL) with early stromal invasion

Fig. 7.**24 b** After application of iodine, the border seen in Fig. 7.**24 a** is accentuated. The leukoplakia is outside the transfor-mation zone. A plaque-like ar-rangement of the keratin is sug-gested

There are good diagnostic criteria to distinguish between the two types, but there is still a gray zone in-between and it is not always possible to categorize a given case as one or the other. Such appearances should always be regarded with suspicion: biopsy should be carried out, or cytology should be repeated. *Fine punctation* characteristically imparts delicate stippling to an otherwise circumscribed grayish-white to reddish area (Fig. 7.26). When the epithelium is keratinized, the dots may appear white, but they are usually red and remain in the same plane as the surface epithelium even after the application of acetic acid. The "dots" in fine punctation are close together (Fig. 7.**23**). Fine punctation is often combined with equally fine mosaic (Fig. 10.**9**). Fine focal punctation may be due to inflam-mation, in which case the margins of the inflamed area appear indistinct after application of iodine (see Figs. 7.**95** and 7.**96 b**). The fine, regular mosaic can also be caused by HPV infection. With the Schiller iodine test, the punctations become yellow to ocher while the adjacent epithelium, due to the koilocytes, stains brown. This is known as iodine-positive punctation (Figs. 7.**26**).

In *coarse punctation*, the petechiae are more pronounced. Not only are they bigger, they are widely separated (Figs. 7.**27**–7.**29**). In extreme cases, punctation appears in the form of papillae; the term *papillary punctation* is then used (Fig. 7.**30**). With higher magnification, corkscrew capillaries can be seen in the papillae. After application of acetic acid, coarse punctation stands out from the plane of the surrounding surface epithelium (Fig. 7.**28 a, b**). Coarse punctation may be com-bined with coarse mosaic. The two patterns may overlap, with intermingling of dots and fissures (Fig. 7.**29**).

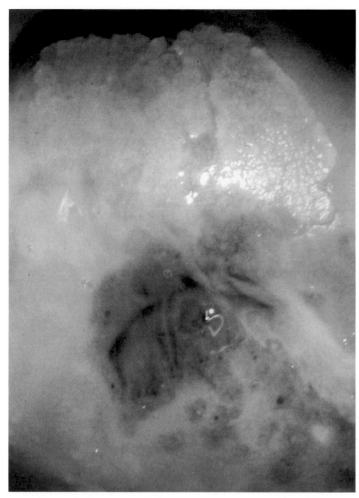

Fig. 7.**25** **Leukoplakia outside the transformation zone,** on the anterior lip. Histology showed acanthotic epithelium

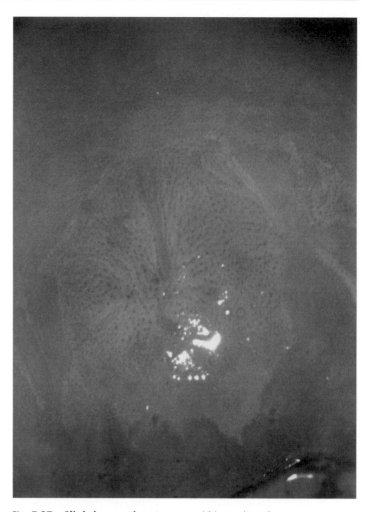

Fig. 7.**27** **Slightly prominent punctation.** The entire, sharply demarcated area apparently lies within unaltered squamous epithelium. Histology showed carcinoma in situ (CIN 3, H-SIL)

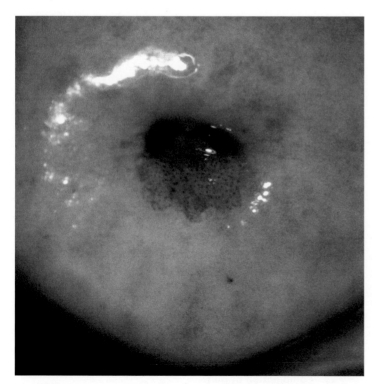

Fig. 7.**26 a** A fine mosaic on the posterior lip of the cervix reaches into the cervical canal. The squamocolumnar junction is not visible

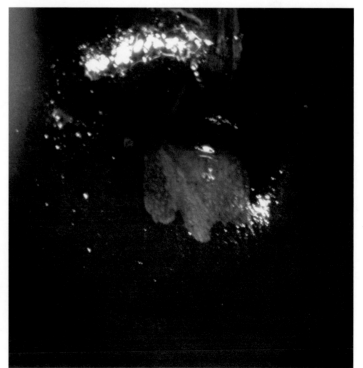

Fig. 7.**26 b** After application of iodine the epithelium is stained brown. This so-called iodine-positive punctation is a sign of HPV infection. Histology showed CIN 1 (L-SIL) with koilocytosis

7.28a

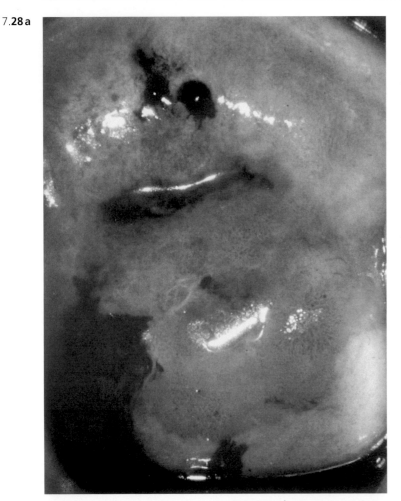

7.28b

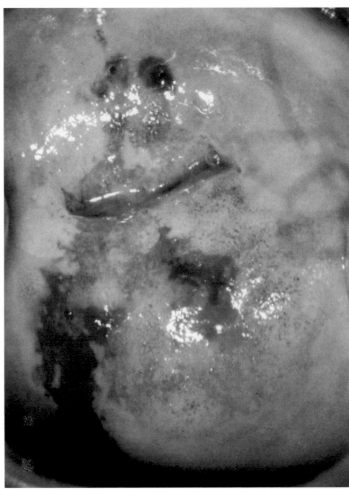

Fig. 7.**28a**   **Atypical yellowish-reddish area** showing focal punctation

Fig. 7.**28b**   After acetic acid application the area of punctation swells, stands out from the surface, and becomes white. Histology showed, carcinoma in situ (CIN 3, H-SIL). An island of fully mature squamous epithelium is seen in the transformation zone on the anterior lip

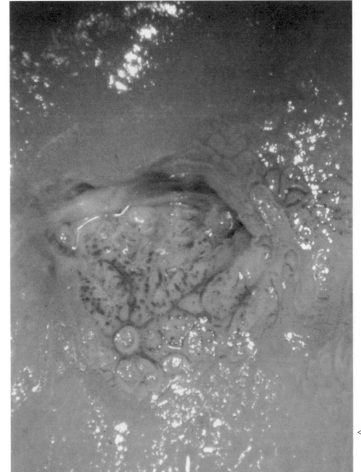

◁ Fig. 7.**29**   **Combination of quite coarse punctation and coarse mosaic.** Histology showed carcinoma in situ (CIN 3, H-SIL)

Fig. 7.**30** **Pronounced papillary punctation.** Histology showed carcinoma in situ (CIN 3, H-SIL) with early stromal invasion

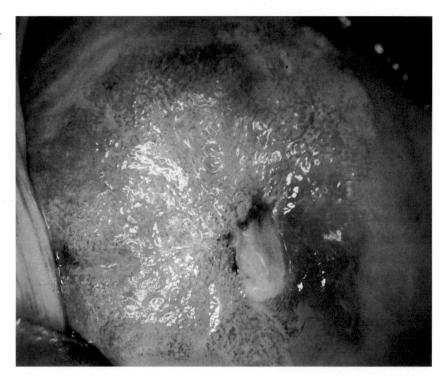

Mosaic

The above remarks about punctation also apply to mosaic. As with punctation, the appearances of mosaic are determined by epithelial changes, which allow distinction between
a) *fine mosaic* and
b) *coarse mosaic.*
Fine mosaic, like fine punctation, occurs in sharply demarcated areas in the plane of the surface epithelium. The appearance of such an area before application of acetic acid can be quite non-specific and can remind one of a relatively vascular transformation zone, which, however, is usually devoid of gland openings or cysts (Figs. 7.**31**–7.**35**, 7.**38**). A distinct color change to gray-white occurs with acetic acid application, and the margins become sharp. The blood vessels become less conspicuous (Fig. 7.**31 b**). The whole area remains in the same plane as before. The mosaic pattern is delineated by the fine network of pale red lines. Such an area may not display the mosaic pattern throughout its entirety; in places, the surface may be uniform and flat because the epithelium is not supported by elongated stromal papillae.

It is often difficult to classify mosaic as fine or coarse (Fig. 7.**36**). Such intermediate forms are mostly caused by lower grade squamous intraepithelial lesions, which may also produce various forms of punctation, depending on the degree of atypia and epithelial architecture.

Coarse mosaic is characterized by greater irregularity of the mosaic pattern. The network of fissures is more pronounced and intensely red. The furrows are more widely spaced, and the epithelial cobbles between them are bigger and more variable in shape than in the fine form (Figs. 7.**34**–7.**38**).

The swelling due to acetic acid makes the structures stand out (Fig. 7.**38**); the peak effect may take a minute to develop. The metamorphosis can be observed before one's eyes as the coarse structure of the mosaic and punctation gradually appears. In contrast, the effect of acetic acid on fine mosaic is immediate.

Hinselmann thought mosaic (which he termed *"Felderung"*) was due to glandular involvement by squamous epithelium (5, 6). Certainly in such cases one can see small white spots that stand out clearly against the reddish background. If the glands (filled with squamous epithelium) are closely packed together, the appearance may simulate a coarse mosaic (Fig. 7.**39**). In such cases the nature of the epithelial plugs in the glands cannot be determined colposcopically and biopsy is recommended.

As mentioned previously, gland openings and nabothian follicles are not usually found within areas of punctation or mosaic. Like leukoplakia, mosaic and punctation can also be found outside the transformation zone, in original squamous epithelium (Figs. 7.**25**–7.**27**, 7.**36**; see also Fig. 7.**52**). This fact is fundamental to the understanding of the morphogenesis of punctation and mosaic as well as to that of epithelial atypia. Punctation and mosaic can occur in isolated fields (Figs. 7.**25**–7.**27**, and 7.**36**) and can coexist with other lesions (see Figs. 10.**1** and 10.**3**). In the latter case the more peripherally located lesions usually represent lower-grade lesions (CIN 1, L-SIL) or merely acanthotic epithelium.

This was confirmed by topographic studies showing that mosaic and punctation occur more commonly outside than inside the transformation zone (84% vs. 16%). Histologically, mosaic and punctation outside the transformation zone corresponded to benign acanthotic epithelium in 70% and to CIN in only 30% of treated cases. Within the transformation zone the respective rates were 20% and 80% (3). In other words, mosaic and punctation within the transformation zone are more likely to represent CIN than the same lesions outside the transformation zone.

7.**31**a

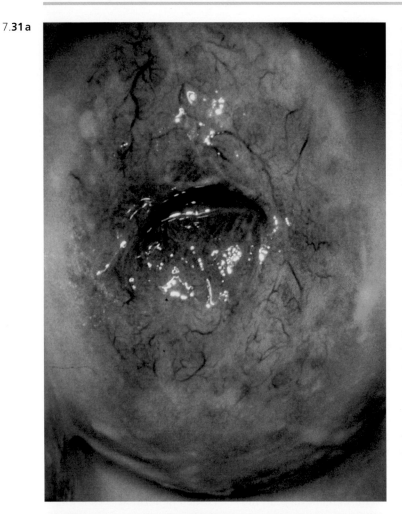

7.**31**b

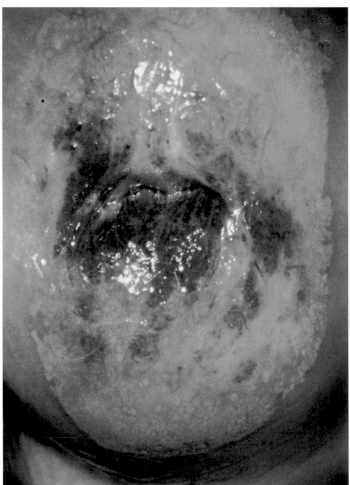

Fig. 7.**31a** **Regularly branching blood vessels in a reddish-yellow, colposcopically atypical lesion** before application of acetic acid

Fig. 7.**31b** **Acetic acid suppresses the vascular pattern,** but brings out a sharply demarcated fine mosaic with a distinct change in color tone. Histology showed acanthotic epithelium

◁ Fig. 7.**32** **Fine mosaic,** mainly on the anterior lip of the external os, after application of acetic acid. Histology showed acanthotic epithelium. The string of an IUD is visible

Fig. 7.**33a** **Indistinct lesion** ▷ outside an intensely red area around the external os. There is increased vascularity on the posterior lip at the edge of the area on close examination

Fig. 7.**33b** **An unexpectedly** ▷ **large, fine mosaic** appears mainly on the anterior lip after the application of acetic acid. The whitish points in the narrow transformation zone are glands filled by squamous epithelium. Histology showed acanthotic epithelium

Fig. 7.**34a** **Transformation** ▷ **zone** surrounded by a semicircular area that turns whitish after the application of acetic acid and shows a clear mosaic

Fig. 7.**34b** Higher magnification ▷ shows that the mosaic is coarser and more irregular than in Figs. 7.**31**–7.**33**. Histology showed CIN 1 (L-SIL)

7.33 a

7.33 b

7.34 a

7.34 b

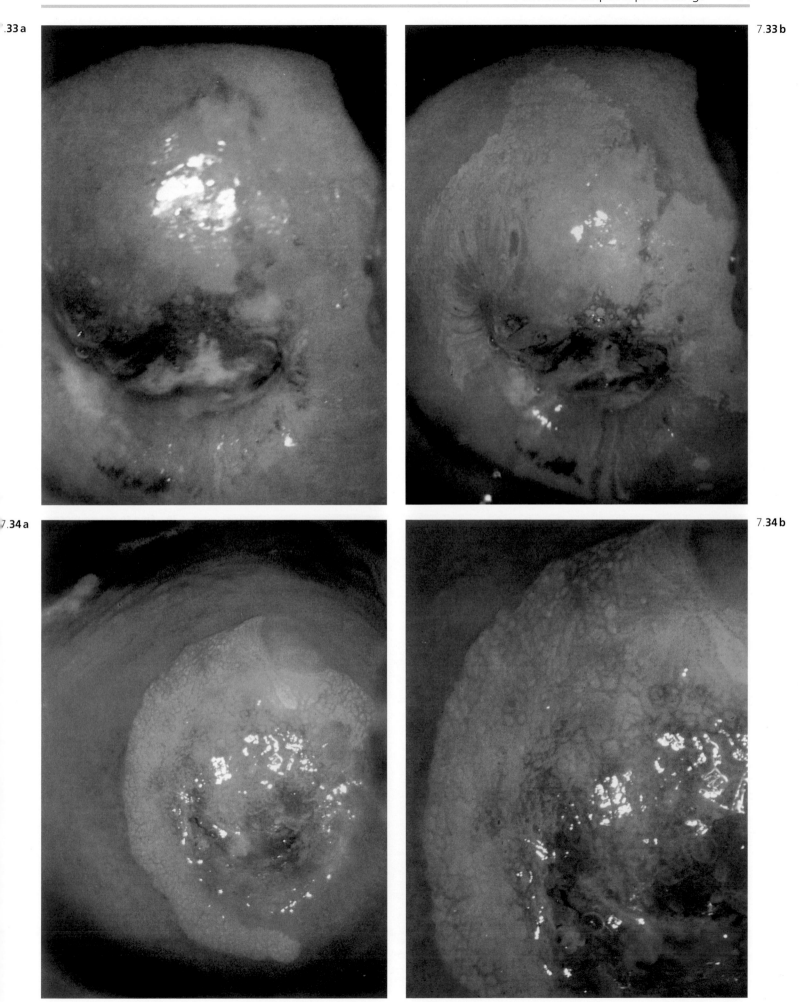

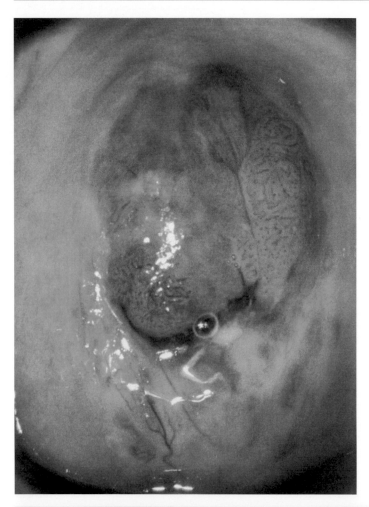

Fig. 7.**35** **Coarse, irregular mosaic** at the edge of a transformation zone after the application of acetic acid. Histology showed CIN 2 (H-SIL). On the anterior lip there is a regular vascular pattern in a mature transformation zone

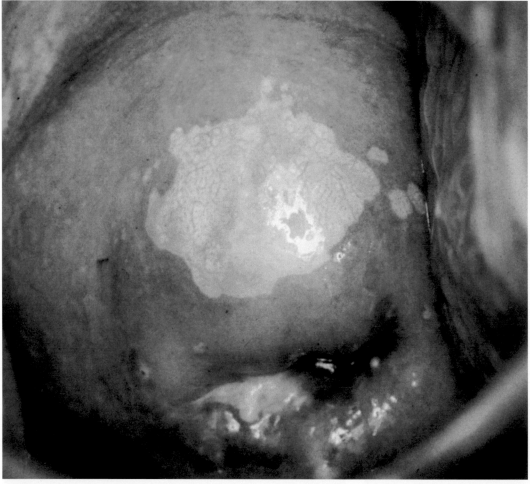

Fig. 7.**36** **Fine to coarse mosaic outside the transformation zone** involving original squamous epithelium. Histology showed CIN 2 (H-SIL)

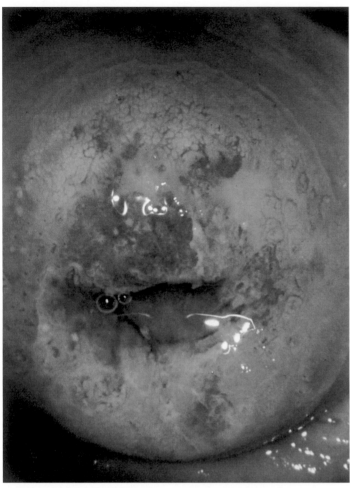

7.38

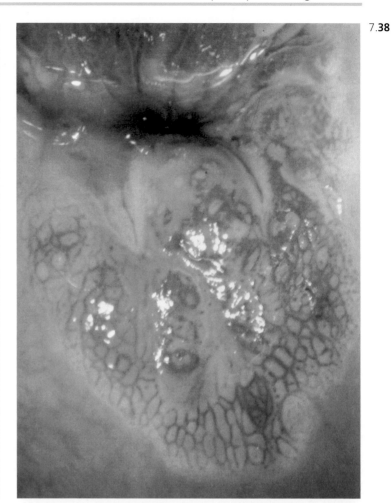

Fig. 7.**37** **Moderately to distinctly coarse mosaic** around the os. Histology showed CIN 3 (H-SIL)

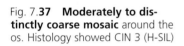

Fig. 7.**38** **Coarse mosaic intermingling with coarse punctation** on the posterior lip. Its border with an unusual transformation zone is sharp. The latter returned carcinoma in situ (CIN 3) and the former severe dysplasia (CIN 3)

7.39

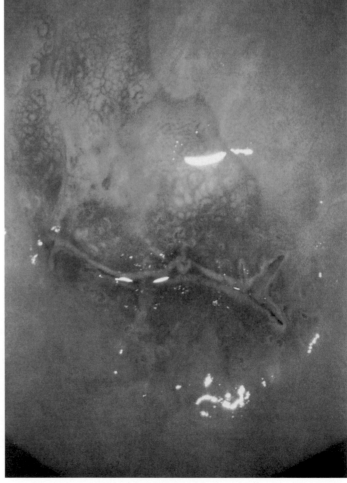

Fig. 7.**39** **Coarse mosaic** at the edge of an unusual transformation zone with cuffed gland openings and solid white points. The points correspond to atypical squamous epithelium in the glands. Histology showed carcinoma in situ (CIN 3, H-SIL)

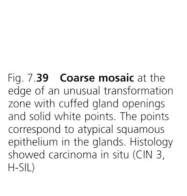

Atypical Transformation Zone

We do not use the term "atypical transformation zone" as an umbrella designation for practically all the abnormal colposcopic appearances such as leukoplakia, punctation, and mosaic, as these also occur outside the transformation zone (Figs. 7.25–7.27, 7.36; see also Figs. 7.52 and 10.3). Naturally, it would be possible to expand the concept of transformation to every type of colposcopic lesion because all atypical epithelia are the result of transformation, whether of columnar or original squamous epithelium. It appears more reasonable to confine the use of the term "transformation zone" to its original context, that is the area where columnar epithelium is converted to squamous. This area is characterized by the presence of ectopy. In contrast, areas of potential change within the squamous epithelium cannot be predicted. Thus, the statement that cervical cancer arises in an atypical transformation zone is fundamentally wrong. To avoid any misunderstanding, we continue to use the term "atypical transformation zone" (2, 4, 15) synonomously with "white epithelium". The designation *"unusual transformation zone"* did not gain wide acceptance.

White epithelium does not show the patterns of mosaic, punctation, or leukoplakia. It does usually contain gland openings, and even retention cysts. It usually corresponds in principle to the normal transformation zone, but differs from it in several important respects. It is characterized, therefore, by the hallmarks of transformation (e.g., gland openings, retention cysts, residual islands of columnar epithelium) but differs from normal in one or more of the following features (2):

1. A dull to yellow-red color before application of acetic acid.
2. A more pronounced color change from red to white with acetic acid application.
3. Cuffed gland openings.
4. A richer vascularity with occasional atypical vessels.
5. A characteristic yellow tinge after application of iodine, with at least part of its circumference being sharply demarcated.

These criteria do not always signify the development of atypical epithelium. Transformation can also result in an acanthotic epithelium with only slight keratinization and no elongated stromal papillae, and thus will not appear colposcopically as keratosis, punctation, or mosaic. When compared to normal, acanthotic epithelium undergoes a more distinct color change with acetic acid, and its junction with original squamous epithelium is sharply defined (Fig. 7.31). In spite of these differences, it is not always possible to distinguish colposcopically between acanthotic epithelium and CIN. Even the whitish epithelium of CIN (H-SIL) may be only discrete, so that it can be difficult to distinguish from a normal transformation zone (Fig. 7.41).

There may be hints of the presence of white epithelium before application of acetic acid. The most difficult to evaluate are the color tones. Any shade of red other than the fresh red of the normal transformation zone should be viewed with suspicion. Grayish red tones, which give the transformation zone an opaque appearance, and yellow shades, which are probably due to marked inflammatory infiltration of the stroma (Figs. 7.42a and 7.45a), are particularly worrisome. In such cases, acetic acid usually induces a distinct white color change and reveals their sharp borders (Figs. 7.42b and 7.45b). A rich vascular bed suggests unusual transformation but is not pathognomonic of epithelial atypia. Only in the presence of atypical vessels arranged in a haphazard manner is such a possibility highly likely (Fig. 7.43).

Actually, the best criterion is the acetic acid test. The more marked the color change and the greater the swelling, the higher the likelihood of epithelial atypia (Figs. 7.44 and 7.45b). However, the spectrum of color changes is wide (Figs. 7.46 and 7.47a).

Fig. 7.**40** **White epithelium (atypical transformation zone)** after application of acetic acid. There are only isolated gland openings. Histology showed carcinoma in situ (CIN 3, H-SIL)

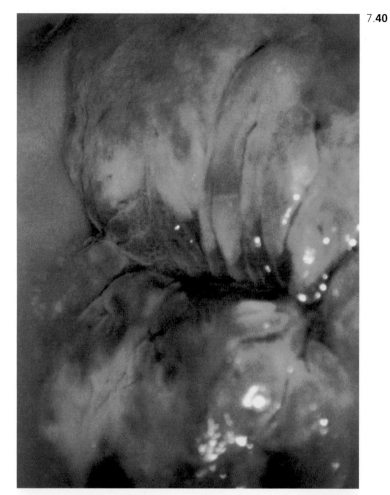

Fig. 7.**41a** **Characteristic appearance of white epithelium (atypical transformation zone)**, distinguished from the typical transformation zone only by the aceto-white epithelium and some cuffed gland openings. There are numerous gland openings. Histology showed CIN 1 (L-SIL)

Fig. 7.**41b** The Schiller test reveals a variegated appearance due to admixture of atypical epithelium and fully mature brown squamous epithelium

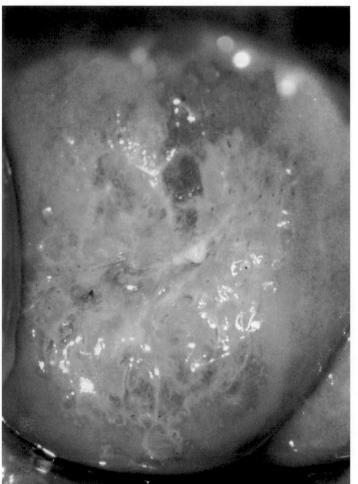

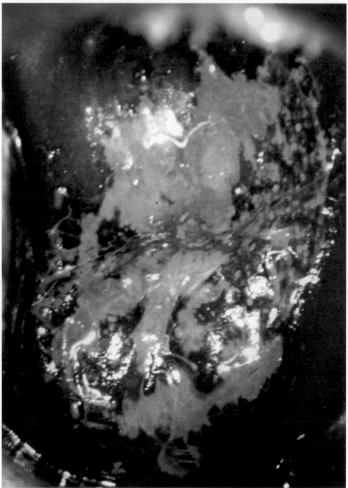

7.**42 a**

7.**42 b**

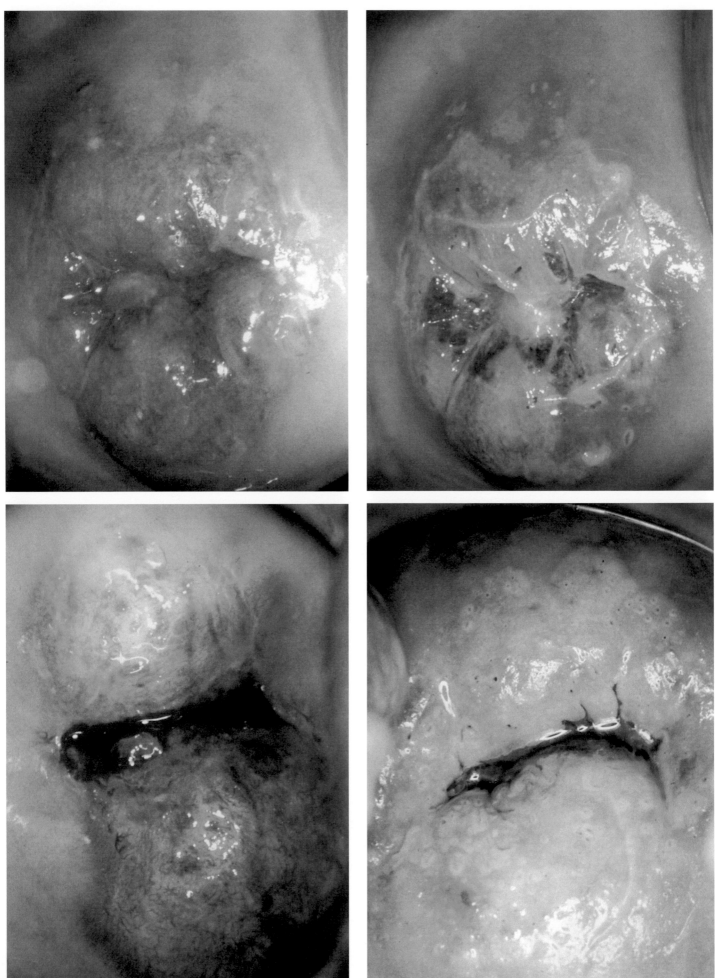

7.**43**

7.**44**

7.45 a

7.45 b

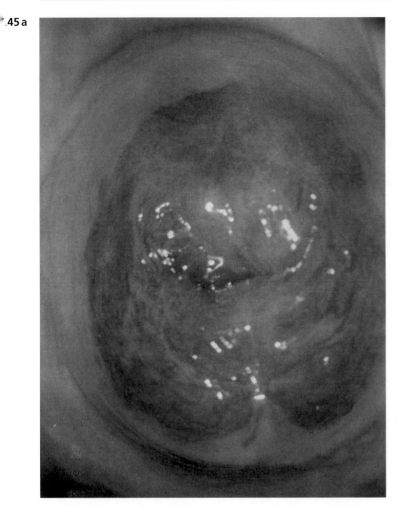

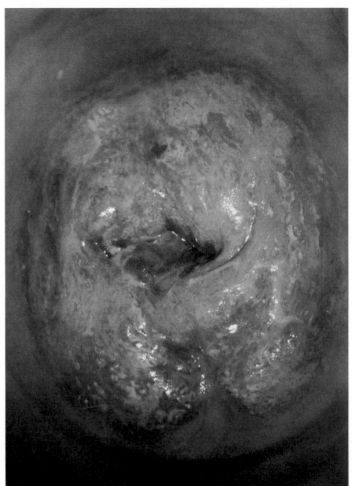

Fig. 7.**45 a** **Angry red transformation zone,** sharply demarcated from the original squamous epithelium

Fig. 7.**45 b** **Patchy appearance** after application of acetic acid. Between the coarse and irregular white patches there are reddish areas with cuffed gland openings and solid epithelial pegs in the glands. Histology showed carcinoma in situ (CIN 3)

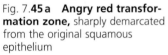 Fig. 7.**42 a** Before application of acetic acid, the white epithelium (atypical transformation zone) is an indistinct grayish red to reddish yellow. Several nabothian follicles shine through the reddish surface epithelium

◁ Fig. 7.**42 b** The white change is produced by acetic acid. Some gland openings are cuffed. The lesion between the 11-o'clock and 12-o'clock positions is due to glandular involvement. Histology showed CIN 1 (L-SIL)

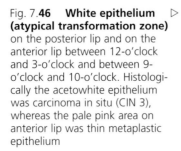 Fig. 7.**43** **Markedly vascular transformation zone** on the posterior lip. Some atypical vessels are seen among the dense vascular network. Histology showed carcinoma in situ (CIN 3)

◁ Fig. 7.**44** **Intense acetowhite epithelium (atypical transformation zone)** with numerous cuffed gland openings. Histology showed CIN 3 (H-SIL)

Fig. 7.**46** **White epithelium** ▷ **(atypical transformation zone)** on the posterior lip and on the anterior lip between 12-o'clock and 3-o'clock and between 9-o'clock and 10-o'clock. Histologically the acetowhite epithelium was carcinoma in situ (CIN 3), whereas the pale pink area on anterior lip was thin metaplastic epithelium

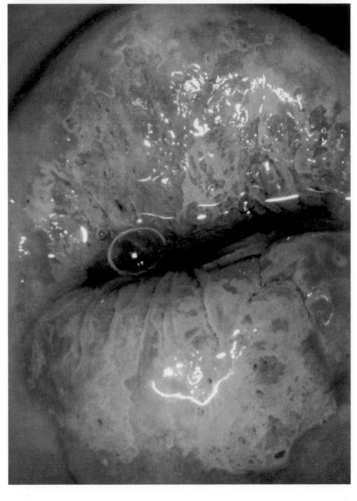

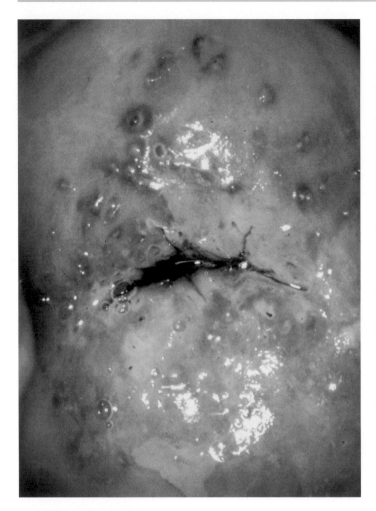

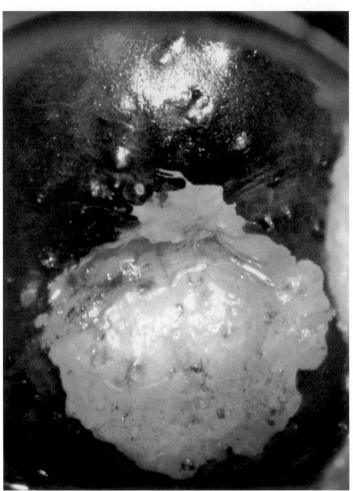

Fig. 7.47 a White epithelium (atypical transformation zone) involving the entire posterior lip as well as the external os between 11-o'clock and 1-o'clock. Note the whiteness of the epithelium and the gland openings, some of which are cuffed. Histology showed carcinoma in situ (CIN 3, H-SIL)

Fig. 7.47 b After iodine staining, the pathologic epithelium clearly stands out against the fully mature squamous epithelium in the transformation zone

Erosion (Ulcer)

The old colposcopic literature used the term *true erosion* because in those days all macroscopically visible lesions of the cervix were designated as erosions. Currently, the term is restricted to cases of epithelial defects. If these are deep, with exposure of the stroma, one speaks of an *ulcer*.

To regard erosion as an abnormal colposcopic finding is correct insofar as ulceration does not occur normally in women of childbearing age. In contrast, the atrophic epithelium of postmenopausal women is prone to develop erosions even during gynecologic examination. Atypical epithelium is particularly vulnerable as it lacks cohesiveness, being more loosely structured than normal squamous epithelium. This feature accounts for the exfoliation of cells detected in smears as well as the swelling induced by acetic acid. The epithelium is also less firmly attached to the underlying stroma, from which it may detach with ease to produce an erosion.

Such ulcers are less easy to see when they occur within a colposcopically evident lesion (Fig. 7.**48**). They are seen better with iodine because the exposed stroma does not stain (Fig. 7.**48 b**). An ulcer can be recognized by its intense red color, its granular floor, and its punched-out margin (Figs. 7.**49**, 7.**50**).

It is even more important not to miss larger ulcers that result from detachment of whole epithelial fields (Fig. 7.**50**). Careful examination of the edges of such defects will reveal residual epithelium, which differs from surrounding normal epithelium by its color and acetic acid reaction. Such residual epithelial rims should always undergo biopsy.

As endophytic carcinomas (Fig. 7.**51**) can masquerade as erosions or flat ulcers, the latter should be probed with a Chrobak's sound (see Fig. 3.**8**). Stroma infiltrated by tumor offers no resistance, the sound advances as into butter. With normal tissues the probe encounters an elastic resistance.

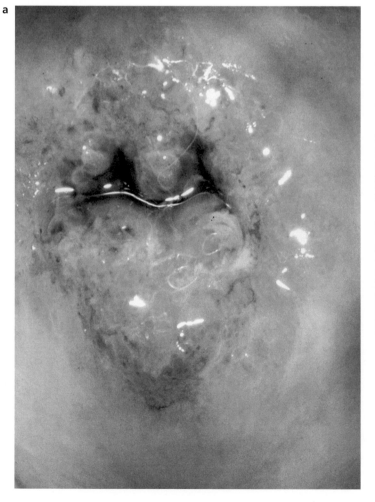

a

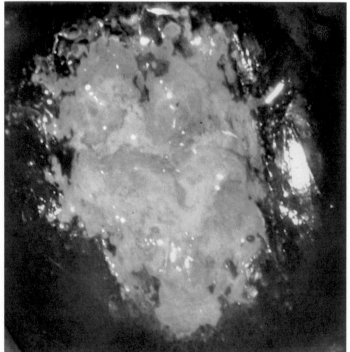

b

Fig. 7.**48 a**   **True erosion at the outskirts of an atypical transformation zone.** The step-like edge, with pathologic as well as normal squamous epithelium, is well shown in places. Biopsy of the whitish epithelium showed CIN 2 (H-SIL)

Fig. 7.**48 b**   After application of iodine, the pathologic epithelium in Fig. 7.**48 a** is typically iodine-yellow, whereas the erosion does not stain at all

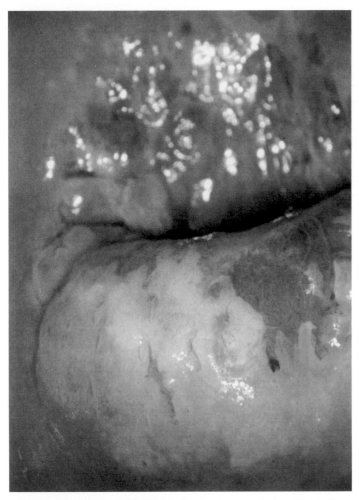

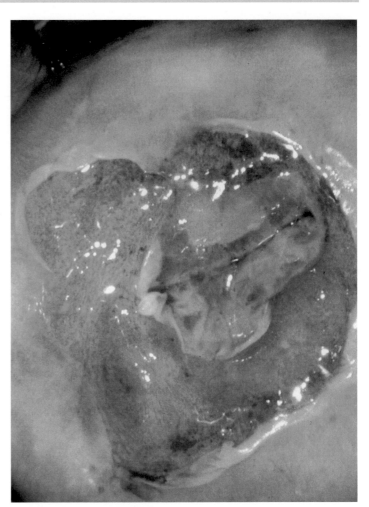

Fig. 7.**49**   **Typical erosion in white epithelium (atypical transformation zone).** The epithelial denudation has revealed the intensely red stroma. Histology of the whitish epithelium showed CIN 3 (H-SIL)

Fig. 7.**50**   **Extensive erosion.** Both toward the endocervical canal and bordering the peripheral normal squamous epithelium, islands of histologically atypical epithelium remain (CIN 3, H-SIL). The texture of the exposed stroma is easily seen

Fig. 7.**51**   **Flat ulcer** to the left of the external os; its floor is uneven and yellowish to dark red. The diagnosis was invasive squamous cell carcinoma

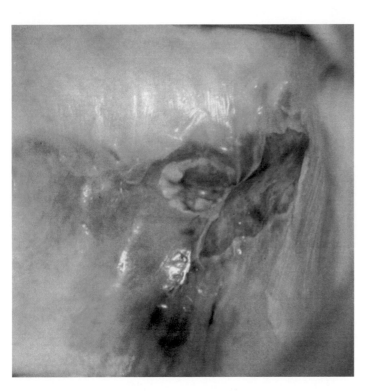

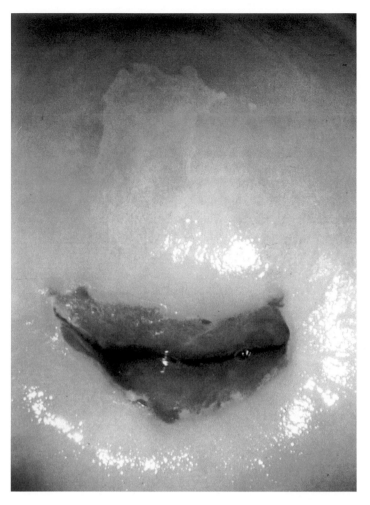

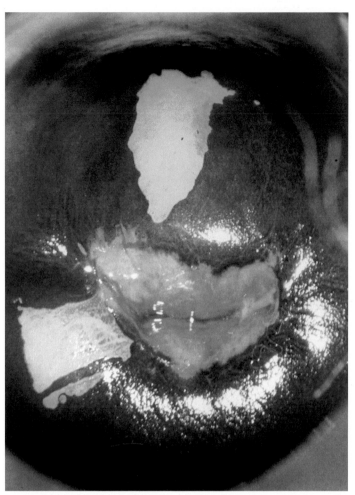

Fig. 7.**52 a**   Only nuances in color suggest a lesion arising in original squamous epithelium. Such a lesion can be easily overlooked during routine colposcopy

Fig. 7.**52 b**   It is remarkable how the above area stands out with its bright yellow color after application of iodine. There is also a second yellow lesion, hardly recognizable in Fig. 7.**52 a**. Histology showed acanthotic epithelium

Inconspicuous Iodine-Yellow Area

If one uses the Schiller (iodine) test at every colposcopic examination, time and again one will encounter sharply circumscribed iodine-yellow areas that are otherwise either not visible or overlooked. Such areas are especially striking if the cervix appears completely normal at first sight (Fig. 7.**52**). If one has the opportunity to re-examine the patient after the iodine reaction has abated or at some later time, the previously iodine-yellow area will appear grayish and sharply demarcated when consciously searched for.

Besides such unsuspected and isolated foci, iodine-yellow areas are also found in combination with other colposcopic lesions; the latter are therefore really bigger and have different outlines than at first suspected (Fig. 7.**53**).

Colposcopically inconspicuous iodine-yellow areas are usually caused by benign acanthotic epithelium. The risk of neoplasia is low (Table 9.**1**).

7.**53**a

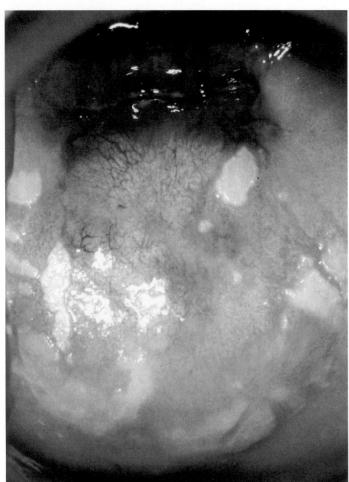

Signs of Early Invasive Carcinoma

Colposcopic detection of small invasive lesions depends on their volume. Foci of early stromal invasion (ESI), which reach only a fraction of a millimeter into the cervical stroma, cannot be seen with the colposcope. Also, such foci arise more often from glands involved by CIN than from atypical surface epithelium. In the latter case, the colposcopic appearance is that of the parent surface epithelium.

The colposcopic signs of ESI are indirect. The likelihood of ESI increases with the surface extent of a lesion. Also, ESI is more common when simultaneously there are different types of epithelia (Table 9.**2**). Some cases show all these features. Increased vascularity also suggests invasion (Figs. 7.**54**, 7.**57**).

Fig. 7.**53 a** **Keratoses** in a vascular transformation zone

Fig. 7.**53 b** It is surprising how brown the vascular epithelium becomes with iodine, whereas the presence of the clearly circumscribed iodine-yellow areas could not be suspected before. Histology CIN 3, H-SIL showed in the transformation zone

Fig. 7.**54** **Markedly vascular transformation zone.**
At the periphery, between 4-o'clock and 6-o'clock, there is a moderately coarse mosaic as well as clearly delineated mild keratosis (arrows). Biopsy from the transformation zone showed carcinoma in situ (CIN 3) with early stromal invasion and acanthotic epithelium at the white plaques

7.**53 b**

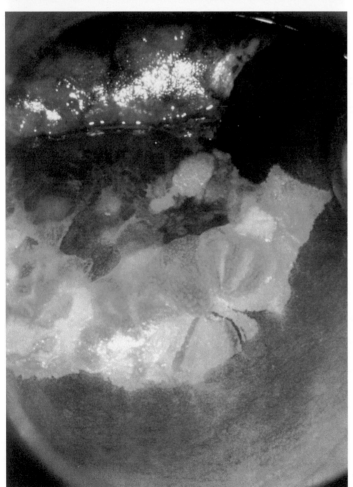

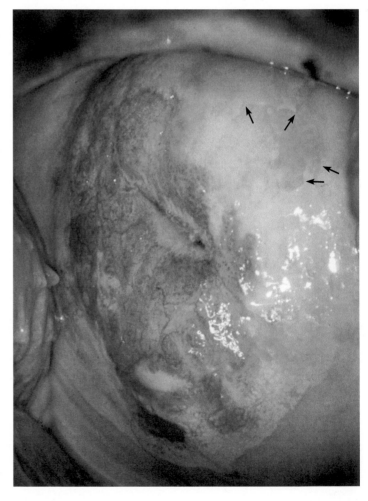

7.**54**

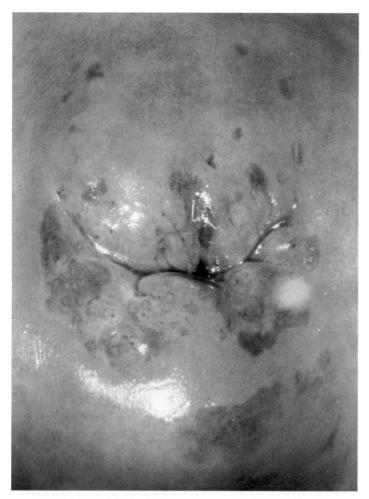

Fig. 7.**55a** **Atypical transformation zone** (white epithelium) that merges imperceptibly with the periphery. Note the separate poorly circumscribed reddish area on the posterior lip

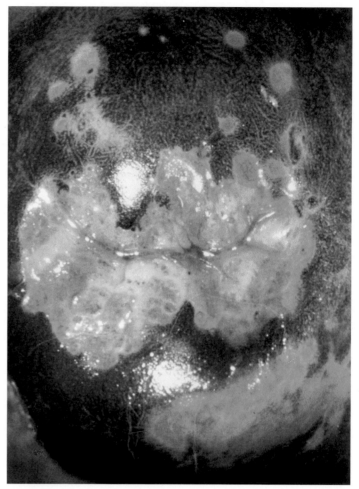

Fig. 7.**55b** The iodine-yellow area around the external os was carcinoma in situ (CIN 3) with early stromal invasion. The isolated area on the posterior lip was inflammatory. The speckled brown lesion on the anterior lip is condylomatous colpitis (see pp. 182, 184)

Although the likelihood of ESI increases with the size of a lesion, quite small or poorly vascularized lesions can be invasive. There are also cases of ESI with a surprising paucity of colposcopic changes (Figs. 7.**55**, 7.**56** and 7.**59**).

Colposcopic detection of *microinvasive carcinomas* depends on their size and location. If a microinvasive carcinoma is entirely within the cervical canal, the ectocervix will show no clue of the lesion. Ectocervical lesions characterized by focal collections of atypical vessels are highly suspicious for microinvasive carcinoma. Atypical vessels are invariably restricted to the invasive focus (Figs. 7.**58**–7.**62**). The vessels are often drawn out, have an irregular course, and are prone to bleed.

Somewhat larger tumors can produce a slight bump on the surface that gives away their location (Figs. 7.**60**, 7.**61**), or they can form a confined polypoid lesion (Fig. 7.**63**). The diagnosis of an invasive lesion arising within an already vascular transformation zone is difficult, if not impossible. Hints of invasion in such cases be sought only retrospectively by carefully correlating the colposcopic findings with the histology of the conization specimen (Fig. 7.**62**).

7.56

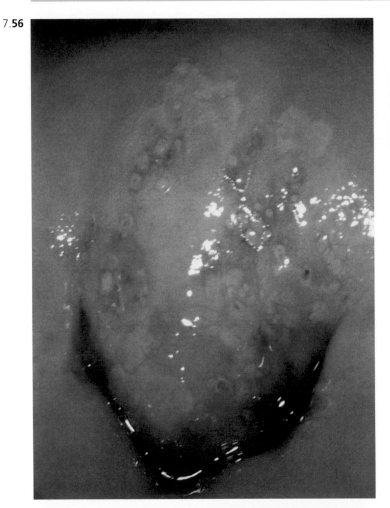

7.57

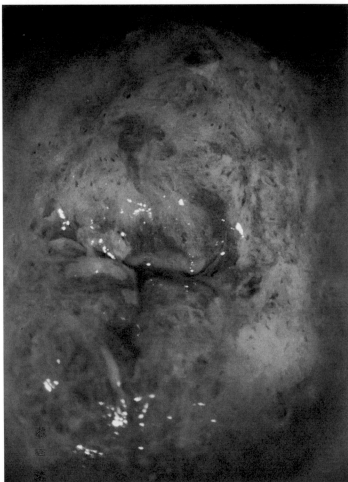

Fig. 7.56 White epithelium (atypical transformation zone) with cuffed gland openings after application of acetic acid. The conization specimen showed carcinoma in situ (CIN 3, H-SIL) with early stromal invasion

Fig. 7.57 White epithelium (atypical transformation zone) with a strikingly coarse surface. In the entire area there are irregularly located, comma-shaped vessels. The conization specimen showed CIN 2, carcinoma in situ (CIN 3, H-SIL), and early stromal invasion

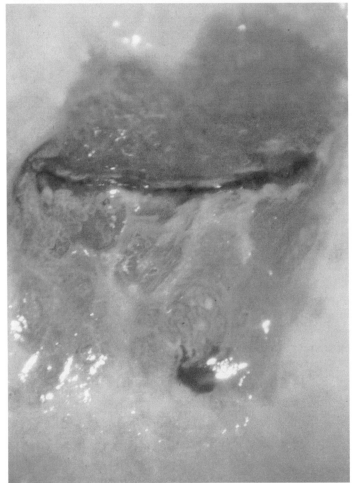

Fig. 7.58 White epithelium (atypical transformation zone), before acetic acid application, harboring a microinvasive carcinoma, just above the bleeding point. Note the irregularly branching vessels. The neighboring reddish areas were carcinoma in situ (CIN 3, H-SIL). True erosion and regenerating epithelium in the vicinity of the external os on the posterior lip and regenerating epithelium on the anterior lip

7.58

Fig. 7.**59** **White epithelium (atypical transformation zone)** after application of 3% acetic acid. Note the friability of the extensive lesion. Histology showed early stromal invasion

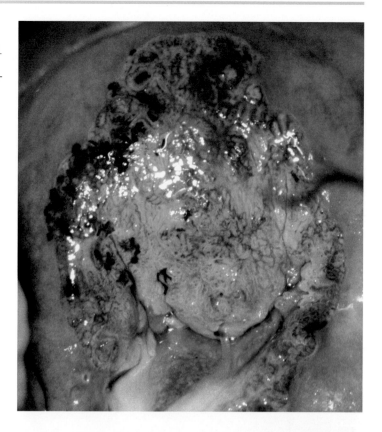

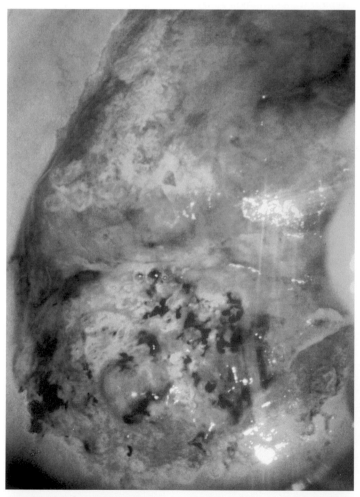

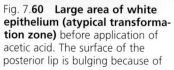

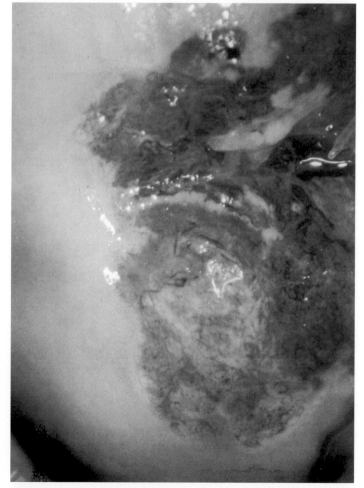

Fig. 7.**60** **Large area of white epithelium (atypical transformation zone)** before application of acetic acid. The surface of the posterior lip is bulging because of the presence of a small invasive carcinoma, no longer a microinvasive carcinoma. Note the extravasation of blood where the vessels are atypical

Fig. 7.**61** **Microinvasive carcinoma** producing a small bulge on the posterior lip. Atypical vessels course over the white surface

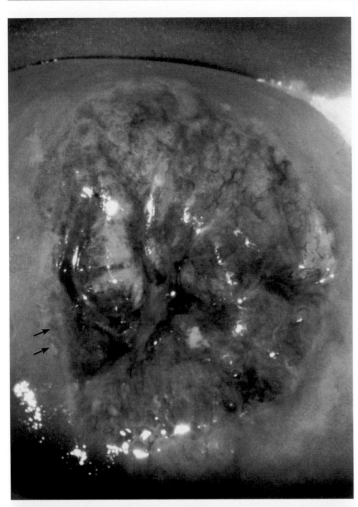

Fig. 7.**62** **Vascular transformation zone** showing focal hemorrhages. The microinvasive carcinoma occupying the left lateral recess of the external os (arrows) is easily overlooked

Fig. 7.**63 a** **White epithelium (atypical transformation zone)** with a coarse surface. The effect of acetic acid is especially marked on the anterior lip: white epithelium with a small polyp in the left corner of the external os

Fig. 7.**63 b** At high magnification the tumor displays numerous atypical vessels. The polyp is a small exophytic carcinoma that has exceeded the limits of a microinvasive carcinoma

7.**63 a**

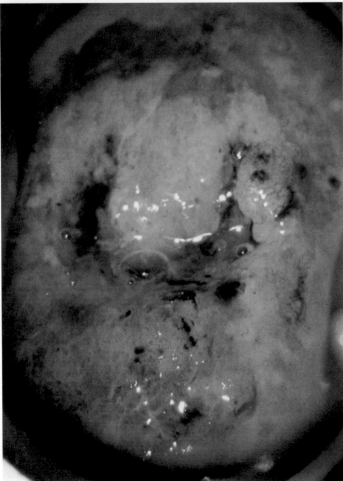

7.**63 b**

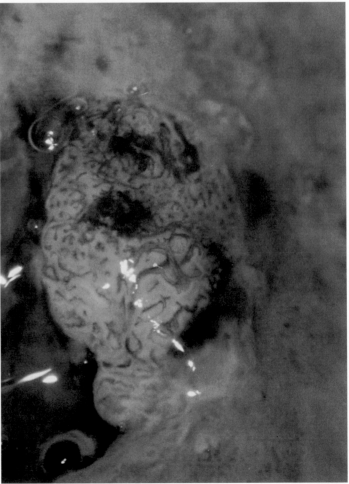

Invasive Carcinoma

(Figs. 7.**64**–7.**74**)

Invasive carcinomas on the ectocervix can be seen with the naked eye. Tumors located entirely within the cervical canal can be seen better with the colposcope, but only if the os is somewhat gaping. In all other cases, colposcopy merely confirms the gross findings.

Distortion of the ectocervical contour depends on the growth pattern of the tumor. Exophytic lesions protrude into the vagina as fungating tumors of varying size (Figs. 7.**64**, 7.**72**). In contrast, purely endophytic neoplasms present merely as red or white eroded areas, the true nature of which can be recognized only by their papillary surface and atypical vessels (Figs. 7.**61**, 7.**73**). Flat endophytic carcinomas with ulcerated surfaces can be difficult to diagnose both with the naked eye and with the colposcope (Figs. 7.**51**, 7.**74**). In such cases, palpation and Chrobak's sound (see p. 17) are of value. Because invasive carcinomas are most often partly exophytic and partly endophytic, their diagnosis should pose no difficulty. Most carcinomas surround the external os (Fig. 7.**66,** see also Fig. 7.**69**). Less often, one or only part of one lip is involved (Fig. 7.**64**).

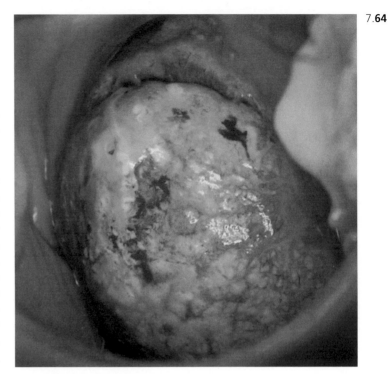

7.**64**

Fig. 7.**64** **Purely exophytic squamous cell carcinoma** on the posterior lip. The tip is ulcerated

Fig. 7.**65** **Exophytic, papillary verrucous carcinoma** around the external os

Fig. 7.**66** **This endophytic invasive squamous cell carcinoma** could be mistaken for white epithelium (atypical transformation zone). The markedly atypical blood vessels on the posterior lip are associated as a rule only with invasive carcinomas

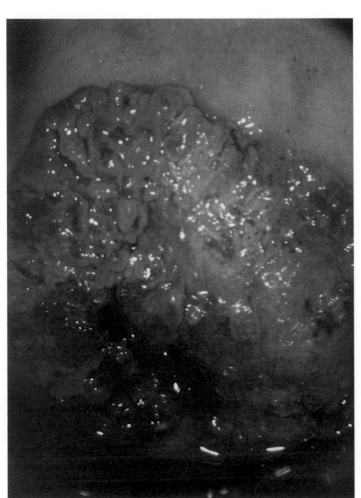

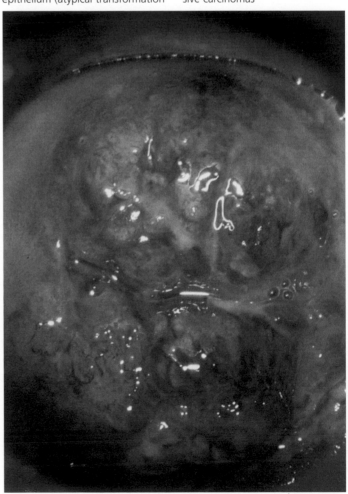

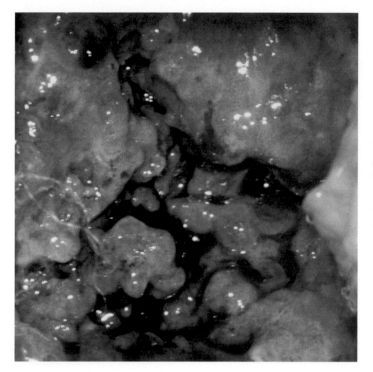

Fig. 7.**67** **Deeply fissured and coarsely papillary invasive squamous cell carcinoma.** The vascular pattern is not pronounced

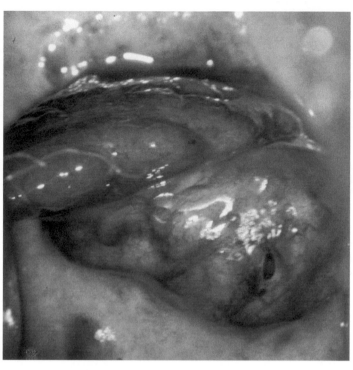

Fig. 7.**68** **Polypoid invasive squamous cell carcinoma,** which could be mistaken for a large benign cervical polyp. The color and blood supply of the polyp lower down are reminiscent of a nabothian follicle

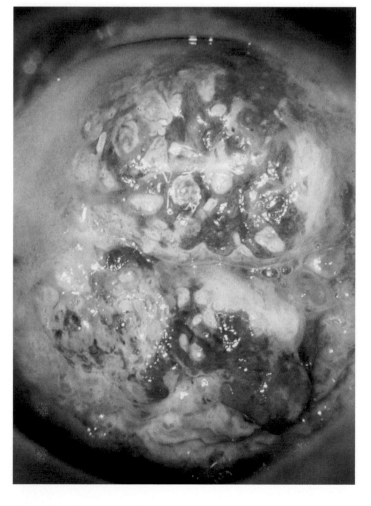

Fig. 7.**69** **Endophytic invasive squamous cell carcinoma** with marked hyperkeratosis

The surface of invasive tumors is usually irregularly fissured (Fig. 7.**67**) like a cauliflower. If the papillae are somewhat finer and more regular, they can be confused with ectopy. The degree of ulceration and tissue destruction is greater in more advanced cancers. Occasionally, tumors present as smooth sessile polyps (Fig. 7.**68**), to be distinguished from benign polyps by their vasculature and by use of Chrobak's sound (Fig. 3.**8**).

An endophytic tumor with a keratotic surface can pose a further diagnostic problem (Fig. 7.**69**). Mistakes can be avoided by always obtaining a biopsy of a keratotic lesion, the nature of which cannot be determined colposcopically because the epithelium is masked by keratin.

7.70a

7.70b

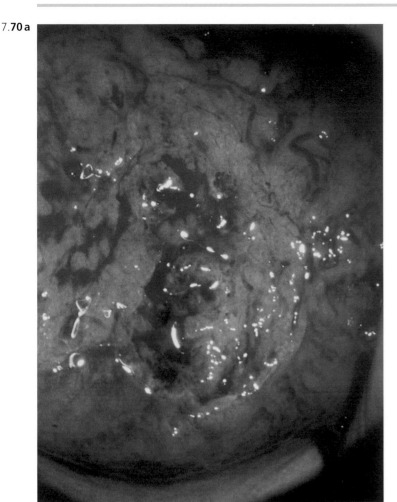

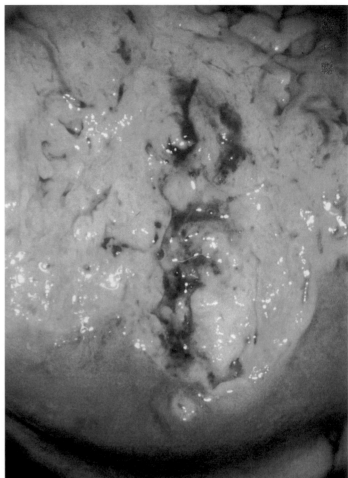

Fig. 7.70a A somewhat ex-ophytic squamous cell carci-noma with a variety of atypical blood vessels

Fig. 7.70b The vascular pattern is suppressed by acetic acid, which turns the background white

Fig. 7.71 Margin of in situ carcinoma around a squamous cell carcinoma that is situated predominantly in the canal. Note the flat ulcer on the anterior lip ▷

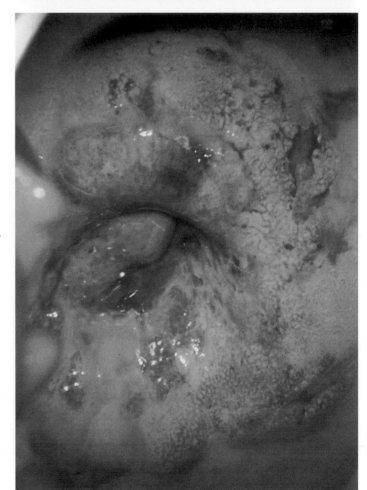

Invasive cancers afford an excellent opportunity to study all kinds of atypical vessels (see p. 121). This should be done after the cervix is cleansed with a dry swab and before applying acetic acid, which makes the vessels blanch (Fig. 7.**70a, b**). Invasive lesions also become more prominent and whitish with acetic acid (Fig. 7.**70**). After the acetic acid test, the criteria for the evaluation of atypical epithelia can be applied to preinvasive lesions, which frequently surround an invasive tumor (Fig. 7.**71**).

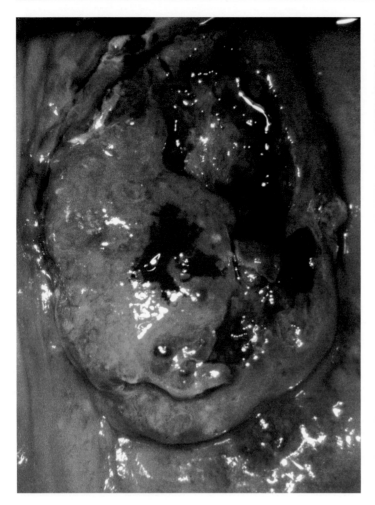

Fig. 7.**72** **Exophytic cervical carcinoma** measuring 4 × 3 cm

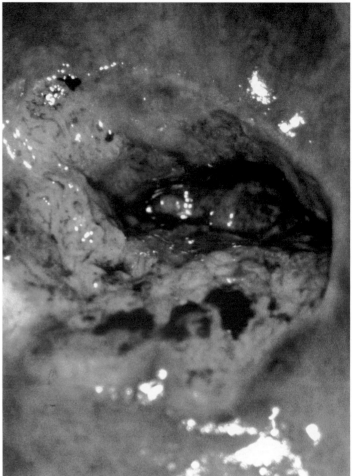

Fig. 7.**73** **Frank invasive squamous cell carcinoma** after application of 3% acetic acid. The vessels are atypical and friable, the surface is irregular

Fig. 7.**74** **Endophytic squamous carcinoma.** Colposcopy shows a patulous external os and leuko-plakia on the posterior lip of the cervix

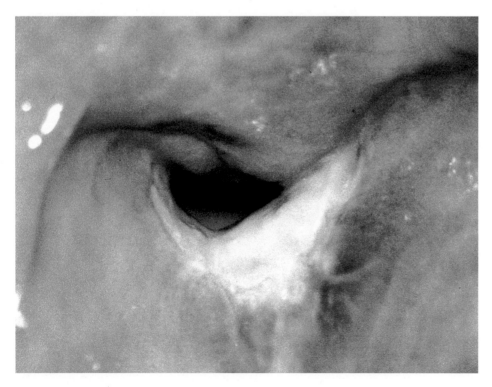

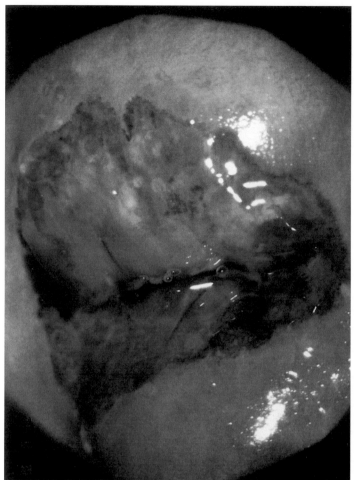

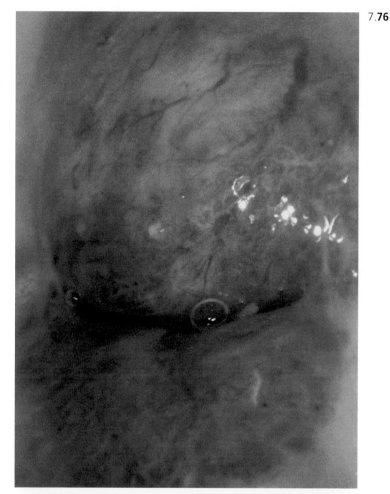

Adenocarcinoma in situ and Microinvasive Adenocarcinoma

There are no colposcopic images that suggest the presence of an adenocarcinoma in situ or of a microinvasive adenocarcinoma (11). Because these lesions usually occur with CIN, one finds the colposcopic changes indicative of CIN (Figs. 7.**75**, 7.**76**). Furthermore, atypical columnar epithelium is usually located in glands or crypts; when on the surface, it is friable and often eroded (Figs. 7.**75** and 7.**77**). The somewhat larger microinvasive adenocarcinoma can occasionally be seen with the colposcope but cannot be distinguished from squamous cell carcinoma at colposcopic magnification (Fig. 7.**77**).

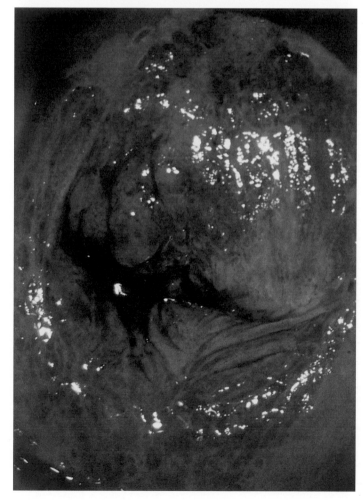

Fig. 7.**75 In this patient with white epithelium (atypical transformation zone) and a suspicious vascular pattern,** the conization specimen showed CIN 1 and 3 (L-SIL and H-SIL) as well as an adenocarcinoma in situ on the ectocervix. The latter was present both in glands and in the superficial columnar epithelium

Fig. 7.**76 Atypical transformation zone** with a few gland opening. Histology showed CIN 2 (H-SIL) on the ectocervix. There is an adenocarcinoma in situ in the lower part of the cervical canal

Fig. 7.**77 Large, partly eroded transformation zone.** The rugae of the everted cervical mucosa are still visible. Histology of the whitish areas showed CIN 2 (H-SIL). On the left side of the cervical os there is a 10×3 mm microinvasive adenocarcinoma

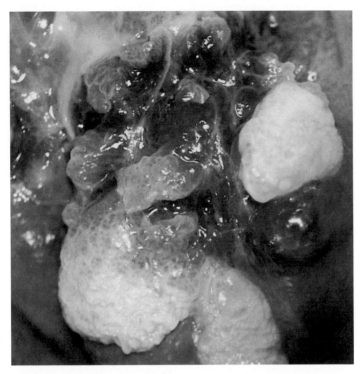

Fig. 7.**78** **Multiple condylomas around the external os.** Only the tips of the large ones show advanced keratinization

Condylomatous Lesions

(Figs. 7.**78**–7.**93**)

Condylomas have attracted a great deal of interest in recent years. The recognition of flat condylomatous lesions on the cervix was crucial for colposcopy, as such changes closely mimic colposcopically suspect findings (8–10) and yet can be reversible and essentially benign. The delineation of condylomatous colpitis (see pp. 88) introduced a new dimension to colposcopic diagnosis, as such changes were previously poorly understood.

Condylomata acuminata are usually easy to diagnose colposcopically. An isolated condyloma in the region of the external os, however, can be mistaken for an exophytic carcinoma (Fig. 7.**78**). Chrobak's sound can be a useful diagnostic aid (see p. 17). The surface of condylomatous lesions is classically papillary (Figs. 7.**78**–7.**80**, 7.**86**, 7.**90**). The structural details, however, can be concealed by keratin, resulting in a smooth, shiny, mother-of-pearl-like surface (Figs. 7.**81**, 7.**85**). Not uncommonly, the papillae are fine and finger-like (Fig. 7.**82**). The color of condylomas varies according to the degree of keratinization and ranges from white and grayish red to intense red.

Fig. 7.**79** **Lacerated external os.** Note the slightly elevated, fine papillary condyloma in a crease, not easily visible to the naked eye

Fig. 7.**80** **Fine papillary condyloma** as an isolated lesion on the anterior lip of the cervix close to the external os. HPV-16 positive. Histology showed a condyloma without atypia

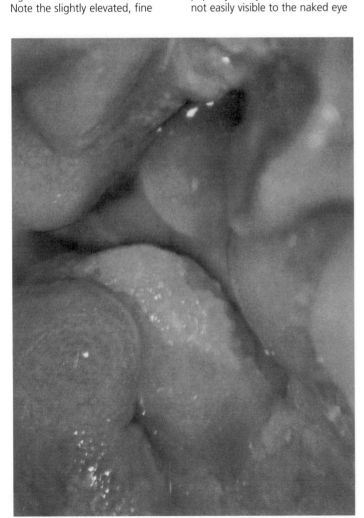

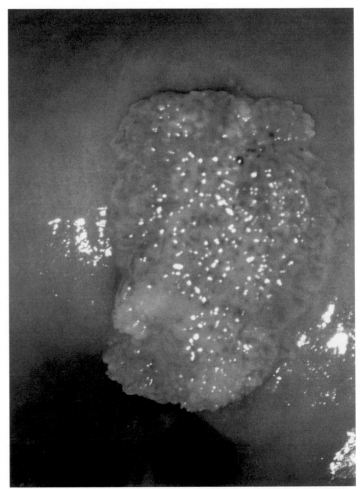

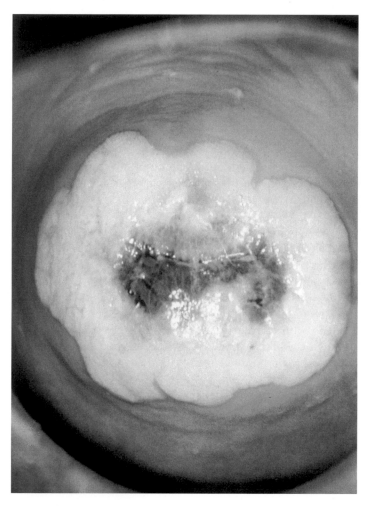

Fig. 7.**81** **Condyloma with marked keratinization.** The keratin layer is so thick that a fissured surface is retained only focally, on the left side

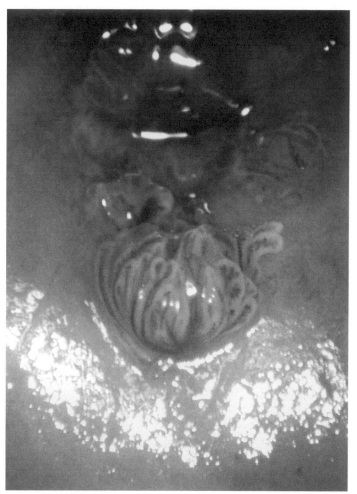

Fig. 7.**82** **Condyloma characterized by finger-like processes** with little in the way of keratinization

Condylomas are often multiple (Figs. 7.**78**, 7.**84**, 8.**9**) and vary in size, providing a good opportunity to study their development. Exophytic condylomas can intermingle with flat lesions (Fig. 7.**84**).

Higher magnification reveals the presence of blood vessels within the papillae of condylomas. They may be comma, corkscrew, or staghorn in shape, and can appear suspicious because of their relatively large caliber (Fig. 7.**83**). Flat and smooth lesions tend to have a distinctive pearly surface as a result of hyperkeratosis (Figs. 7.**84**, 7.**85**). No criteria have been described to distinguish colposcopically between typical and atypical condylomas (10). It is conceivable, however, that the latter may have a coarser structure that may produce coarse punctation or mosaic in analogy with CIN (SIL) and acanthotic epithelium.

The Schiller test shows that condylomatous cells still contain various amounts of glycogen. A stippled, variegated appearance can be produced by focal keratinization (Figs. 7.**86b**, 7.**87**). There is also no difference between infection with different HPV types. To distinguish between condylomatous and non-condylomatous lesions of similar appearance, Reid et al. (13) proposed a grading classification which would suggest subclinical HPV infection. However, other authors found this classification unsatisfactory (12).

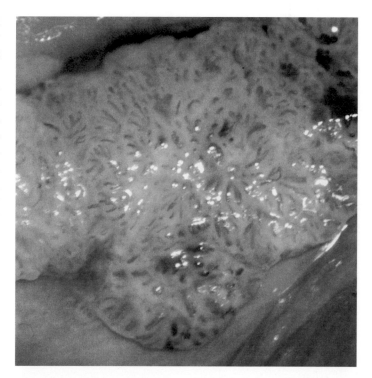

Fig. 7.**83** On higher magnification, the vessels within the papillae are comma-shaped and antler-like. Their coarseness gives the impression of atypicality

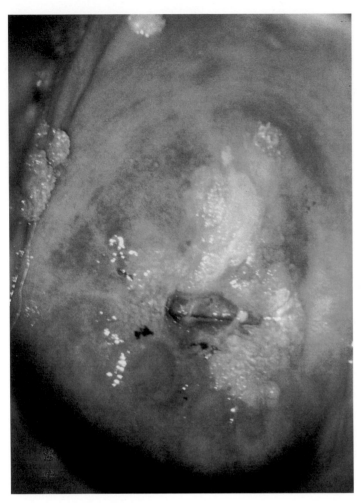

Occasionally, the degree of glycogen storage by condylomatous epithelium produces the hitherto undescribed colposcopic appearance of *iodine-positive mosaic or punctation* (Fig. 7.**89**). It is unclear whether this picture is typical of and always due to condylomatous lesions. At any rate, such mosaic is caused by glycogen-containing epithelium associated with tall stromal papillae. Histologically, the epithelium in such cases is not merely a variant of normal, but shows features suggestive of flat condylomas. An iodine-positive mosaic pattern can be produced by colposcopic lesions that, before the Schiller test, appear nonspecific apart from their pearly surface. The result of the Schiller test in such cases is all the more surprising (Fig. 7.**91**).

Condylomatous lesions frequently coexist with CIN (SIL), in which HPV can usually be found (Figs. 7.**88**–7.**90**).

Experienced colposcopists will have come across an essentially normal cervix and vagina, the surfaces of which are evenly studded with numerous white dots (Fig. 7.**93**). These correspond to the tips of elongated stromal papillae that perforate a rather irregular-structured yet glycogen-containing epithelium. Meisels et al. (10) called this appearance *condylomatous cervicitis and vaginitis.*

Fig. 7.**84**   **Flat condylomas** around the external os. Most of their surface is finely granular, some areas are smooth. HPV-16 and HIV-positive. Small condylomatous lesions dot the cervix and the vagina

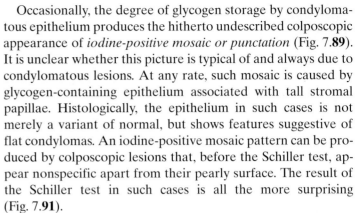

Fig. 7.**85**   **Markedly keratinized flat condyloma** surrounding the external os. Note the characteristic pearly, flat surface

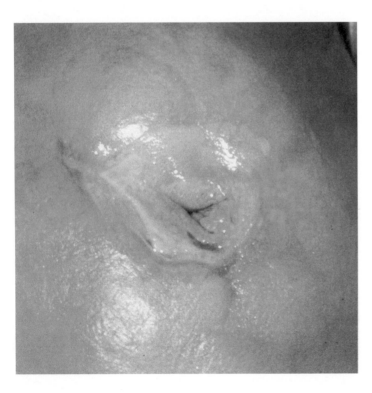

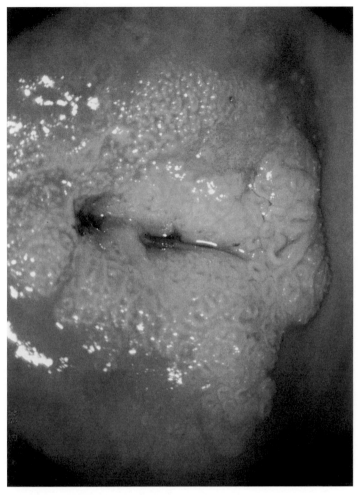

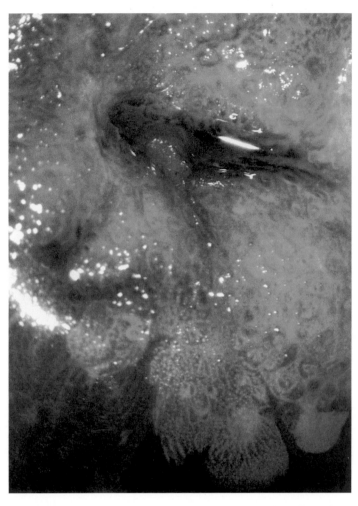

Fig. 7.**86 a   Flat to distinctly elevated condylomas** around the external os and in the lower cervical canal. The same patient as in Fig. 7.**84**, six months later

Fig. 7.**86 b**   The Schiller test shows the typical patchy brown areas indicating glycogen storage in the condylomas. Histology showed CIN 1 (L-SIL) with koilocytosis

Fig. 7.**87   Condyloma.** The brownish color with iodine of glycogen containing patches within the condyloma correlates well with the histologic picture

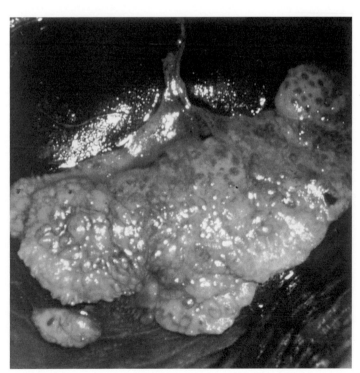

7.88 a

7.88 b

7.89 a

7.89 b

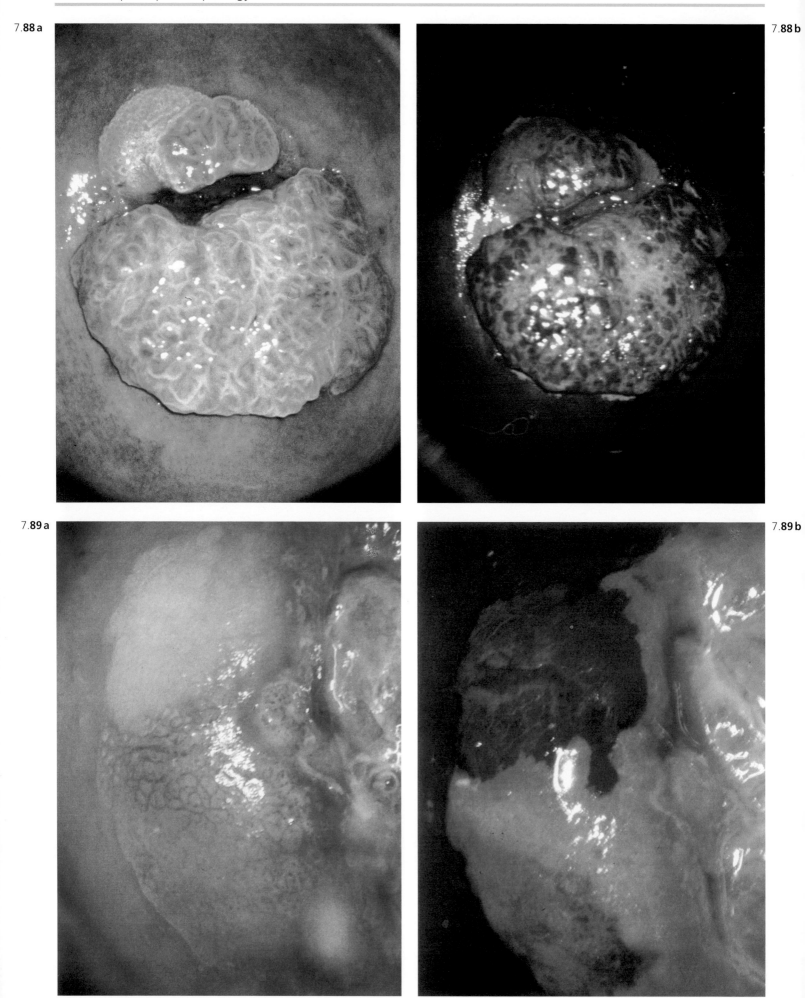

◁ Fig. 7.**88a** **Exophytic condylo-matous lesion** after application of 3% acetic acid **b** After application of iodine the surface shows the patchy brown staining typical of condylomas and an ocher epithelium

◁ Fig. 7.**89a** **A shiny mother-of-pearl surface of a lesion** also showing moderately coarse mosaic and punctation: histologically, the white area corresponded to a flat condyloma, the mosaic showed CIN 1 (L-SIL)

◁ Fig. 7.**89b** The previously white lesion displays an iodine-positive mosaic pattern after the Schiller test: histology showed flat condyloma. The mosaic and punctation, clearly visible before the Schiller test, stain poorly. Less structured areas are light brown

Fig. 7.**90** **Flat, fine papillary condylomatous excrescences within a mosaic field.** The mosaic is HPV-16 positive and histology showed CIN 1 (L-SIL) ▷

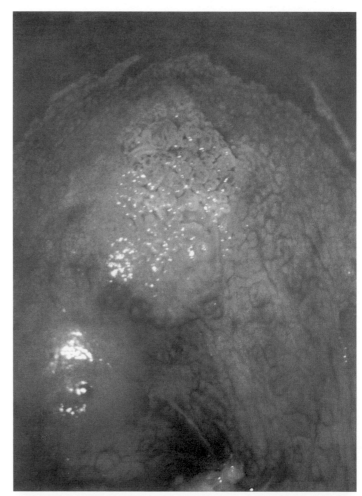

Fig. 7.**91a** **Flat condyloma**

Fig. 7.**91b** The Schiller test reveals an iodine-positive mosaic

7.**91a**

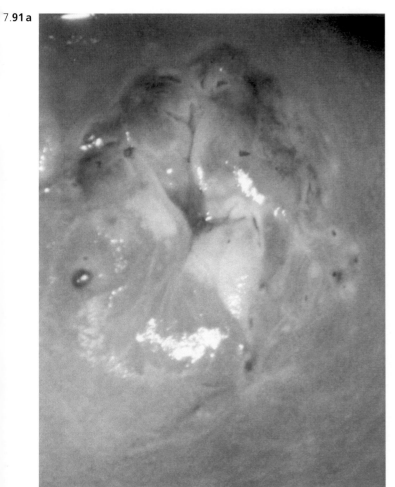

7.**91b**

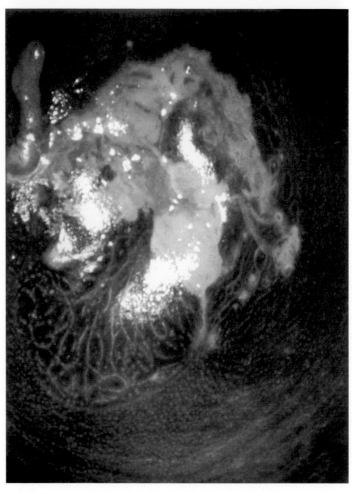

7.92

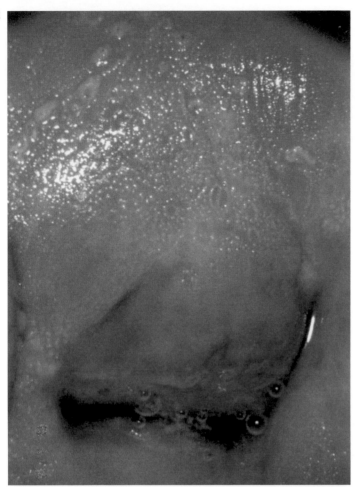

Miscellaneous Colposcopic Findings

Inflammatory Changes

Diffuse inflammation of the vagina has a nonspecific colposcopic appearance. The appearance of focal lesions is of some significance, due to patchy inflammatory infiltration of the stroma accompanied by dilated capillaries. Diagnostic difficulties arise when such foci become bigger and indiscriminately arranged.

Trichomonal infection produces a typical frothy discharge. Removal of the secretions may reveal numerous red spots covering the cervix (Fig. 7.**94a**). The inflammatory foci vary in shape and in distribution. After application of acetic acid, the previously red areas turn whitish, the squamous epithelium being already "loosened up" by the inflammation (Fig. 7.**94b**). The damaged epithelium can release its glycogen, with consequent failure to stain with iodine. Iodine typically imparts a leopard-skin appearance to inflammatory lesions (Fig. 7.**95**) and confirms the poor circumscription of larger ones which may otherwise be mistaken for more serious abnormalities.

Colpitis macularis (strawberry cervix) has a unique colposcopic appearance, characterized by uniformly arranged red spots a few millimeters in size; it is usually due to *Trichomonas vaginalis* (Fig. 7.**96a**). The inflamed area is always iodine-negative, and its margin is indistinct (Fig. 7.**96b**). In severe cases, the vagina is also involved.

7.**93**

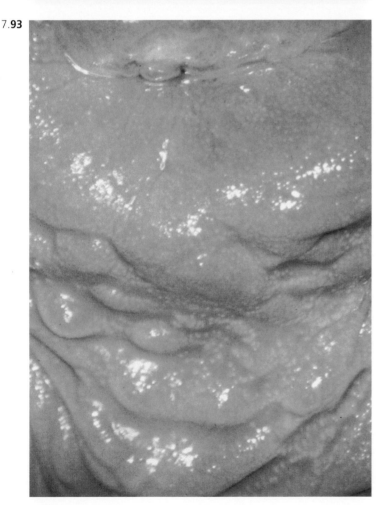

Fig. 7.**92 Typical appearance of the cervical mucosa** in a patient with condylomatous vaginitis. There are circumscribed, slightly elevated condylomas whithin the granular area

Fig. 7.**93 Condylomatous colpitis.** The cervix and the vagina are covered with numerous white spots

94 a

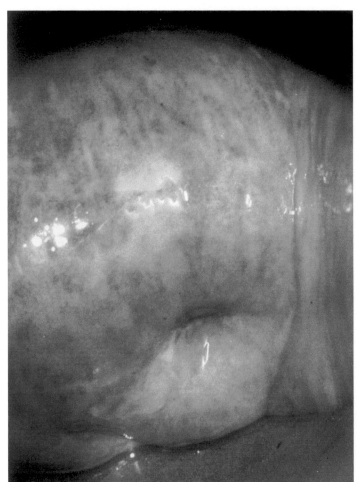

7.94 b

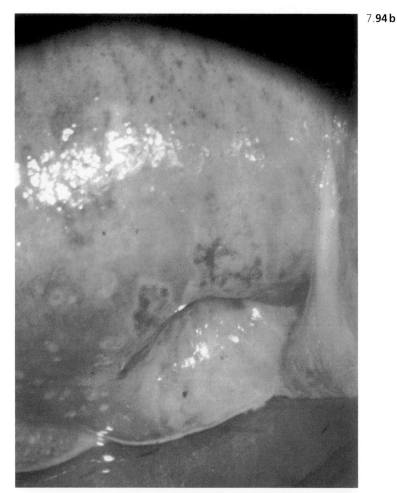

Fig. 7.**94 a** **Irregular reddish stippling of the cervix** due to trichomonas infection

Fig. 7.**94 b** The inflamed area becomes white to some extent after application of acetic acid; its margins are indistinct

7.95

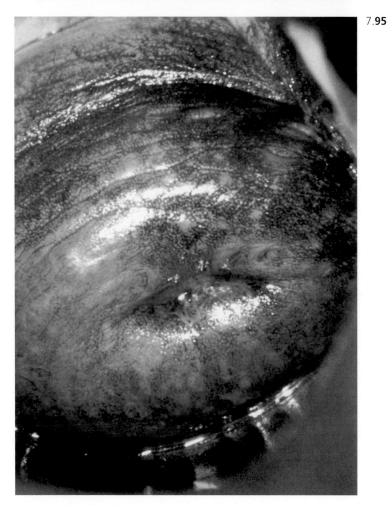

Fig. 7.**95** **The vague margins of the inflamed areas** are well seen with the Schiller test

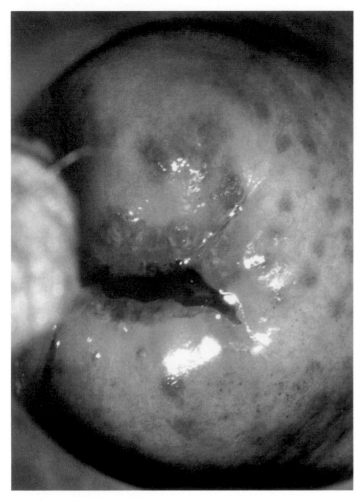

Fig. 7.**96 a** **Colpitis macularis**
(strawberry cervix). Numerous
round spots cover the cervix and
vagina, due to focal round cell infiltration

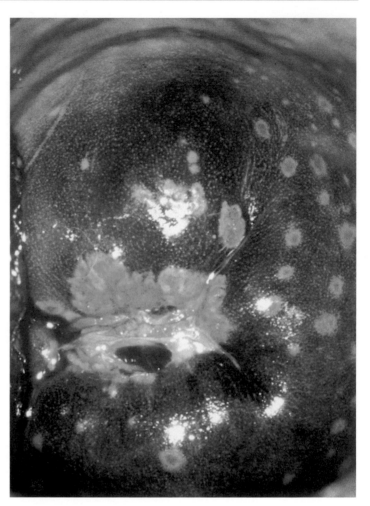

Fig. 7.**96 b** After the Schiller test,
the inflamed areas in Fig. 7.**96 a**
are poorly demarcated and are
separated by fields showing so-
called condylomatous colpitis

Polyps

Polyps are easily seen colposcopically, even if they are situated
farther up in the endocervical canal. The aim of colposcopy is
to detect them and evaluate their surface configuration according to the usual criteria. In the first instance, a polyp can be in-
vested by columnar epithelium only, in which case the typical
grape-like appearance will be seen. More often, the polyp is
covered by smooth squamous epithelium (Figs. 7.**97** to 7.**100**).
If the maturation of such histogenetically metaplastic
squamous epithelium is irregular, then the various fields are
clearly demarcated from each other (Figs. 7.**98**, 7.**101**). Rarely,
the squamous epithelium is atypical; in such cases, the colposcopic changes conform to those that occur elsewhere on the
cervix. Polyps can be single or multiple, and can arise from ec-
topies, from transformation zones (Figs. 7.**97**, 7.**101**, **7.102**), or
from otherwise unremarkable cervices (Fig. 7.**99**). On occasion, bleeding polypoid structures protruding from the cervix
can represent endometrial carcinoma (Fig. 7.**103**) or a myoma
in statu nascendi (Fig. 7.**104**).

7.**97**

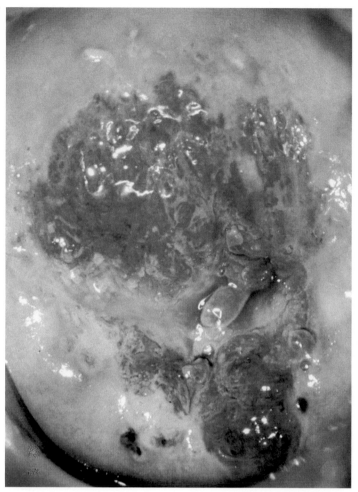

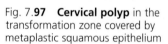

7.**98**

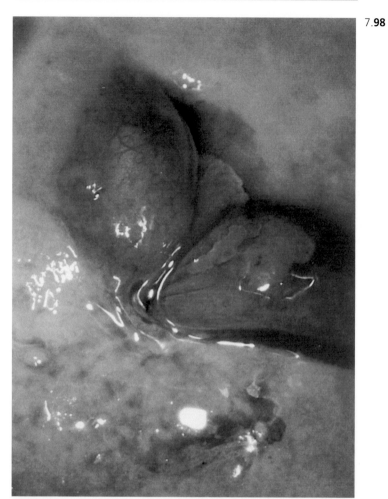

Fig. 7.**97** **Cervical polyp** in the transformation zone covered by metaplastic squamous epithelium

Fig. 7.**98** **Endocervical polyps** that have undergone metaplasia. A nabothian follicle has developed within one of the polyps. The lowermost polyp shows that the metaplastic process developed in separate, well-defined fields

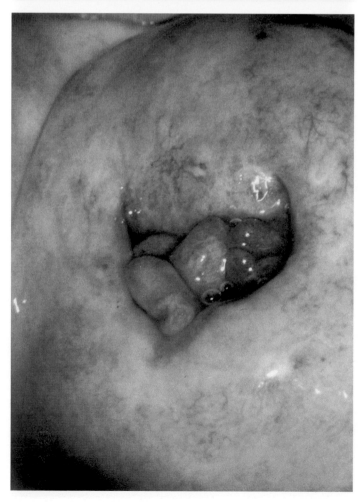

Fig. 7.**99** **Multiple polyps arising from an atrophic cervix.** The metaplastic epithelium covering the polyps also arose in separate fields

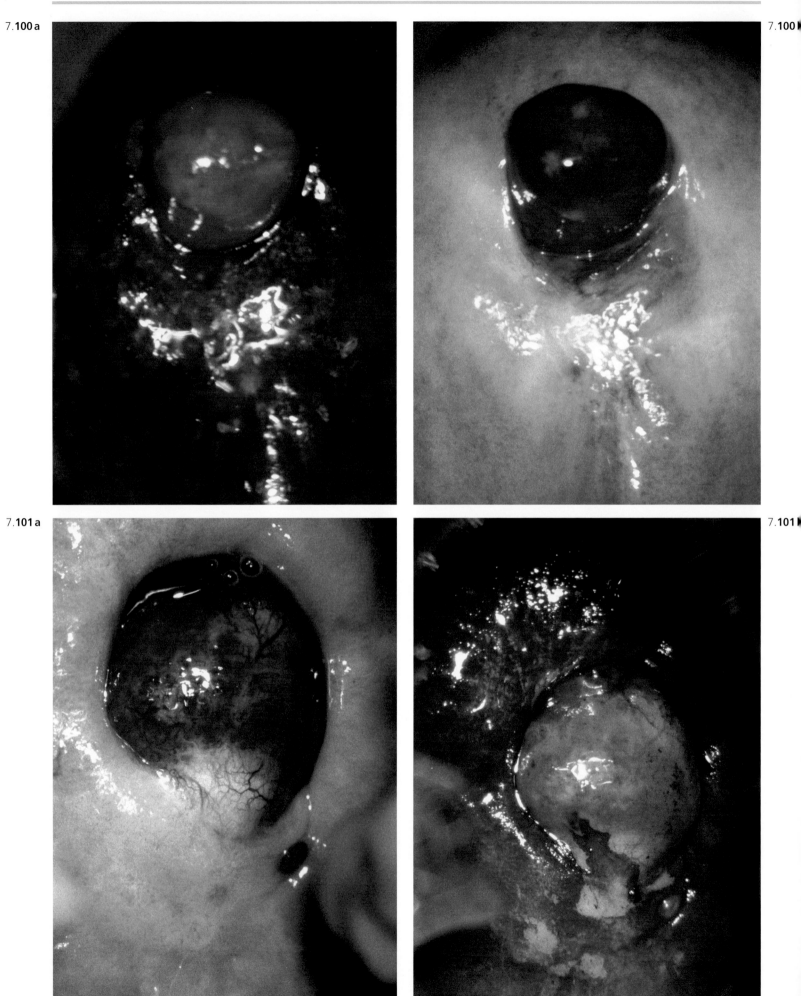

◁ Fig. 7.**100a** **Polyp** protruding from the external os. The surface is smooth and the origin unclear **b** After application of iodine (Schiller test), the cervix stains brown while the polyp stains yellow. Histology showed a cervical musosal polyp with acanthotic epithelium on its surface

◁ Fig. 7.**101a** **Broad-based polypoid structure** corresponding to a nabothian follicle **b** After application of iodine the cervix stains brown and the nabothian follicle yellow

Fig. 7.**103** **Bleeding polyp** protruding out of the cervical canal. The surface of the cervix shows signs of atrophy. Histology showed a FIGO stage IA G1 endometrial carcinoma

7.**103**

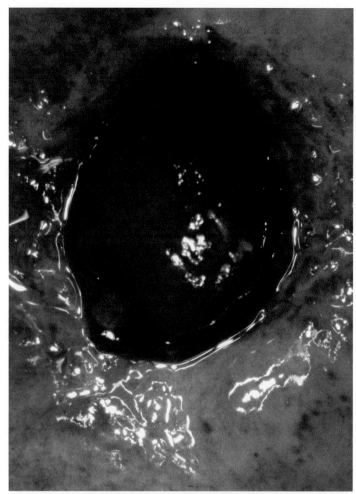

Fig. 7.**102** **Nabothian follicle** with delicate nonsuspicious vessels on its surface

Fig. 7.**104** **Bleeding, polypoid structure** protruding from the external os. The clinical impression was that of a myoma in statu nascendi, histology confirmed a benign leiomyoma

7.**102**

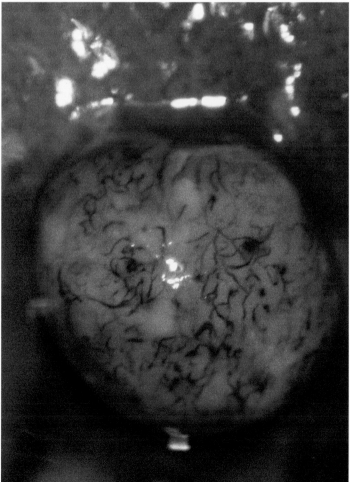

7.**104**

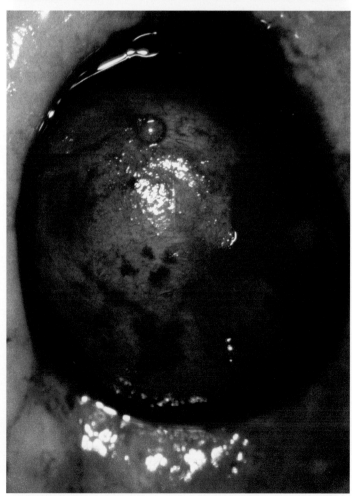

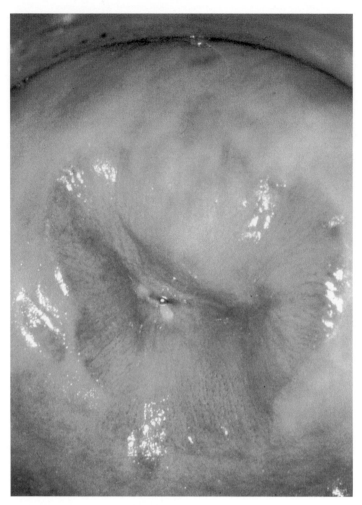

Fig. 7.**105 a**   **Cervix after conization.** The site of surgical removal
can be identified by the scarring
and the fine vasculature

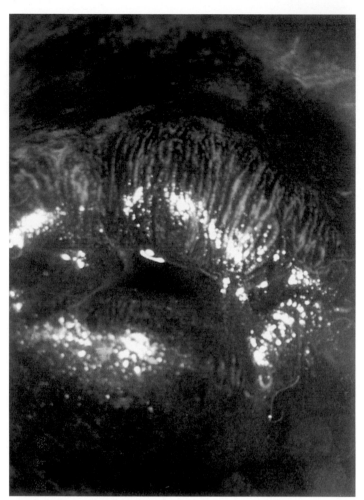

Fig. 7.**105 b**   Iodine staining reveals the uniform nature of the
epithelium. The light yellow streaks
correspond to scars

Postconization Changes

After conization the cervix is usually smooth and covered by
normal squamous epithelium. The squamocolumnar junction
is again situated at the external os. Occasionally the scar after
conization clearly stands out from the residual cervix
(Fig. 7.**105 a**) and can be mistaken for some other abnormality.
But with the Schiller test the region in question stains brown
like the rest of the cervix (Fig. 7.**105 b**), any nuance in color is
due to scar tissue under the epithelium. This is a good example
of how the stroma can influence the colposcopic appearance.
Six weeks after conization scarring can be extensive
(Fig. 7.**106**).

The changes after loop conization are the same after cold-
knife procedures. With correct technique the entire squamocolumnar junction is usually visible, which is helpful for follow-
up colposcopy (Figs. 7.**107**, 7.**108**). Similarly, laser vaporization
techniques have excellent cosmetic results.

Residual lesions due to incomplete excision by conization
can be detected at follow-up colposcopy in the region of the re-
constituted external os (Fig. 7.**110**).

Sturmdorf sutures for hemostasis after conization are considered obsolete, partly because of the poor cosmetic result.

7.106

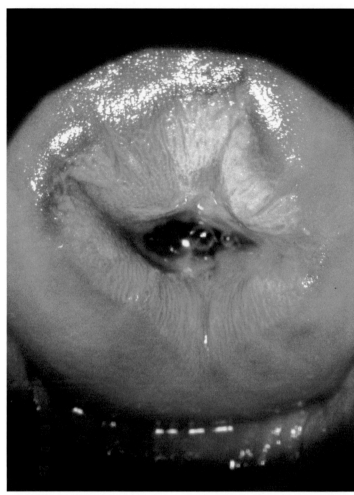

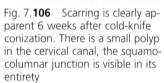

7.107

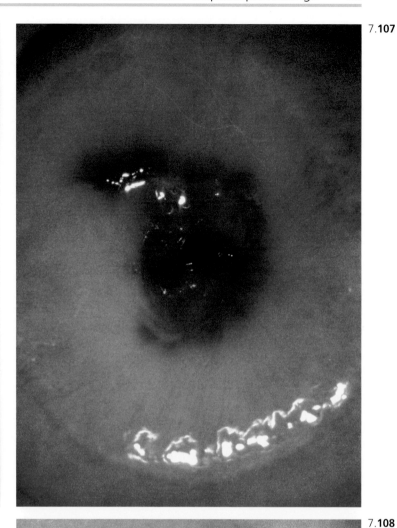

7.108

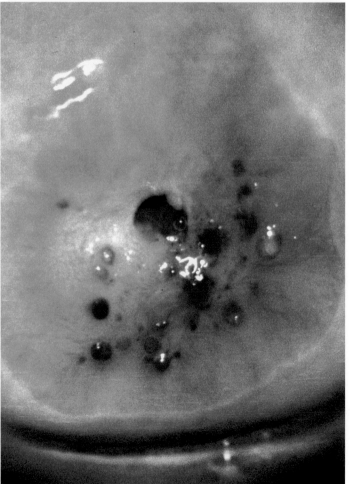

Fig. 7.**106** Scarring is clearly apparent 6 weeks after cold-knife conization. There is a small polyp in the cervical canal, the squamocolumnar junction is visible in its entirety

Fig. 7.**107** A small scar can be seen 6 weeks after loop excision. The squamocolumnar junction is visible in its entirety

Fig. 7.**108** Six weeks after loop excision there is slight scarring on the external os with somewhat increased scarring between 3 and 7 o'clock. Cervical glands with non-suspicious vessels can also be seen

7.**109**

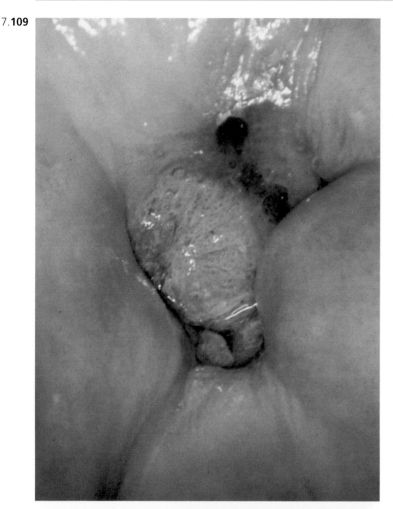

7.**110**

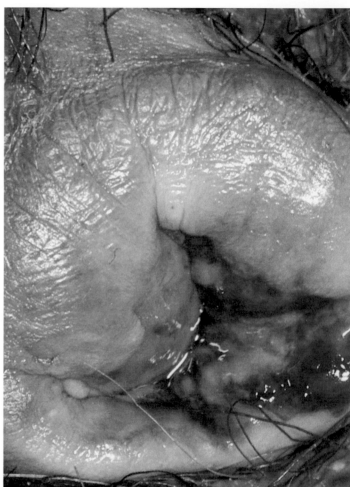

7.**111**

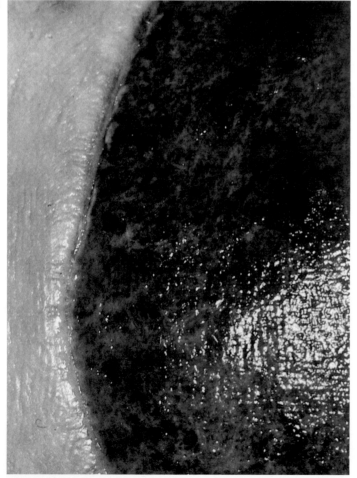

Fig. 7.**109   The cervix following incomplete excision of carcinoma in situ** (CIN 3) by conization. Note among the scar tissue an area of coarse punctation due to residual atypical epithelium

Fig. 7.**110   Typical appearance following epidermization of prolapse.** The ectocervical epithelium assumes the character of wrinkled skin: this is due to various degrees of keratinization

Fig. 7.**111   Part of a decubitus ulcer associated with prolapse.** Note its typically flat floor and punched-out margin

Changes Due to Prolapse

Prolapse results in exteriorization of the squamous epithelium of the cervix and portions of the vagina so as to become part of the body surface. The glycogen-containing squamous epithelium changes and becomes skin-like. Histologically, there are acanthosis and hyperkeratosis.

This process proves that, according to demand, the nonkeratinized glycogen-containing epithelium can become like the epidermis. We call this *epidermization*. As this type of epithelium is not native to the site, the term *abnormally maturing* has been used. Glatthaar (4) referred to it as the *reactive form* of abnormally maturing (acanthotic) epithelium. This produces a diffuse uniform cover, as seen especially in cases of prolapse. Colposcopically, we encounter far more often the *regenerative form* of acanthotic epithelium that arises from metaplasia in clearly defined fields and is of great colposcopic significance. The important difference between the reactive and regenerative types is the reversible nature of the former: after the

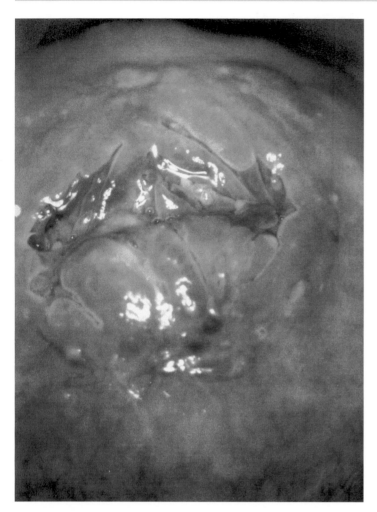

Fig. 7.**112** **Small bluish focus of endometriosis** on the anterior lip of a transformation zone with still   recognizable rugae of the ectropion

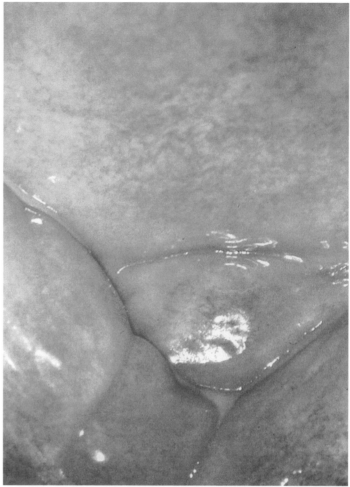

Fig. 7.**113** **Bluish endometriotic deposit** in the posterior fornix of a   38-year-old woman, on day 24 of the cycle

stimulus ceases, i.e., after reduction of the prolapse, the epithelium resumes its original form. The well-circumscribed regenerative type of acanthotic epithelium, on the other hand, retains its position and contour. The regenerative type of acanthotic epithelium therefore is abnormal and in this respect resembles chronic dermatoses.

The colposcopic appearance of the epidermized cervix is reminiscent of skin both in color and in its wrinkled surface contour (Fig. 7.**110**). It is obvious even with the naked eye that this type of epithelium is more durable and less vulnerable. A well-recognized complication of prolapse is ulceration of the extruded portion of the cervix or vagina, known as *decubitus ulcers*. These ulcers are punched out, their floor is flat and usually an angry red (Fig. 7.**111**), but it can be dirty gray if superinfected.

Endometriosis and Miscellaneous Findings

Endometriosis of the cervix is rare (Fig. 7.**112**). The posterior vaginal fornix is involved more frequently (Fig. 7.**113**). The deposits appear as bluish spots shimmering through the epithelium and are best seen before menstruation; they can disappear altogether during the proliferative phase of the cycle.

Fistulas (Fig. 7.**114**), and anatomic anomalies (Fig. 7.**115**) can on occasion be documented at colposcopy.

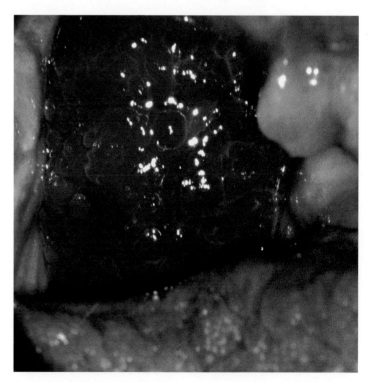

Fig. 7.**114** **Vesicovaginal fistula** after primary radiation treatment for carcinoma of the cervix. The   bladder mucosa is red and grapelike without the application of acetic acid

7.**115a**

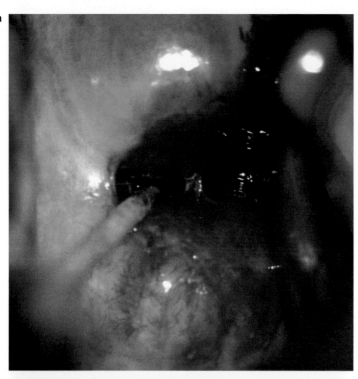

7.**115b**

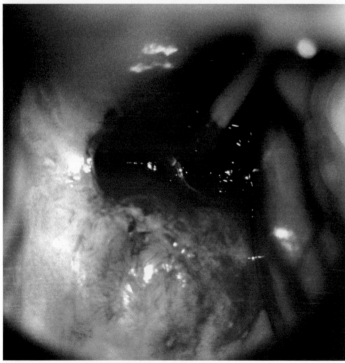

Fig. 7.**115 Transformation zone in a cervix divided by a septum.**
The probe is in the left (**a**) and right (**b**) part of the cervical canal

References

1 Baader O. Kolpophotographische Studien, 1: Die Portio von Adoleszentinnen. Gynäkol Praxis 1982;6:101.

2 Burghardt E. Über die atypische Umwandlungszone. Geburtshilfe Frauenheilkd 1959;19:676.

3 Girardi F. The topography of abnormal colposcopy findings. Cervix 1993;11:45–52.

4 Glatthaar E. Studien über die Morphogenese des Plattenepithelkarzinoms des Portio vaginalis uteri. Basel: Karger, 1950.

5 Hinselmann H. Die Ätiologie, Symptomatologie und Diagnostik des Uteruscarcinomas. In: Veit J, Stöckel W, eds. Handbuch der Gynäkologie, vol. 6:1. Munich: Bergmann, 1930:854.

6 Hinselmann H. Die Kolposkopie. Wuppertal: Girardet, 1954.

7 Hinselmann H. Kolposkopische Studien, vols 1–6. Leipzig: VEB Thieme, 1954–59.

8 Meisels A, Fortin R, Roy M. Condylomatous lesions of the cervix, 2: cytologic, colposcopic and histopathologic study. Acta Cytol 1977;21:379.

9 Meisels A, Morin C, Casas-Cordero M, Roy M, Fortier M. Condylomatöse Veränderungen der Cervix, Vagina und Vulva. Gynäkologe 1981;14:254.

10 Meisels A, Roy M, Fortier M, et al. Human papillomavirus infection of the cervix: the atypical condyloma. Acta Cytol 1981;25:7.

11 Östör AG, Pagano R, Davoren RAM, Fortune DW, Chanen W, Rome R. Adenocarcinoma in situ of the cervix. Int J Gynecol Pathol 1984;3:179.

12 Pixley EC. Colposcopic appearances of human papillomavirus of the uterine cervix: In: Syrjänen K, Gissmann L, Koss LG, eds. Papillomavirus and human disease. Berlin: Springer, 1987:268–295.

13 Reid R, Stanhope CR, Herschman BR, Crum CP, Agronow SJ. Genital warts and cervical cancer, 4: a colposcopic index for differentiating subclinical papillomaviral infection from cervical intraepithelial neoplasia. Am J Obstet Gynecol 1984;149:815.

14 Townsend DE. The cervix and vagina of women exposed to synthetic nonsteroidal oestrogens. In: Coppleson M, Pixley E, Reid B, eds. Colposcopy. Springfield, IL: Thomas, 1978:14–341.

15 Treite P. Die Frühdiagnose des Plattenepithel-Karzinoms am Collum uteri. Stuttgart: Enke, 1944.

8

Colposcopy in Pregnancy

At least one colposcopic examination should be performed during pregnancy, ideally at the time the pregnancy is confirmed. Normally, this will be during the first half of the first trimester. As with nonpregnant patients, a smear should be taken at the same time. A colposcopically suspect lesion can be safely biopsied during the first trimester, and one should proceed as in the nonpregnant patient. Should there have been no gynecologic check-up in the years preceding the pregnancy, it would be a mistake to let another 40 weeks go by without assessing the cervix. If this rule is observed, detection of cervical cancer during the later stages of pregnancy or the puerperium will be avoided.

Pregnancy-Induced Cervical Changes

Pregnancy-related changes in the cervix have been described in detail by Stieve (10) and Fluhmann (3). Colposcopically, the most prominent features are the increase in size and number of the blood vessels and lymphatics, leading to hyperemia of the cervix. The stroma becomes softened and edematous, and enlarged. The endocervical mucosa is hyperplastic. Proliferation of the columnar cells leads to enlargement and complex ramification of the glandular crypts, with the formation of numerous secondary clefts and tunnels (3). The endocervical mucosa thus becomes more plush, due to deeper extension into the stroma. The end result is a honeycomb appearance of the glandular field.

A characteristic change is a *decidual reaction of the stroma*, which can be limited and focal or quite extensive and can even produce polypoid lesions referred to as "decidual polyps" (Figs. 8.**9**–8.**11**).

The concept of "erosion" during pregnancy is controversial. Colposcopically, this corresponds to ectopy, with or without signs of a transformation zone. The frequency of this finding in advanced pregnancy (3) has led to the supposition that it is due to prolapse of the mucosa during the second half of the pregnancy (6). According to Fluhmann (3), erosions during pregnancy may be preexistent, evolve during pregnancy, or come about during labor. Coppleson and Reid (1) found that both erosions and subsequent squamous epithelial metaplasia occur especially during the first pregnancy. In later pregnancies, there were no major changes. We are unable to support this view.

In our experience, an ectocervix completely covered by squamous epithelium need not undergo any change during the course of the pregnancy. It is also possible to produce "pseudo-erosion" during the later stages of pregnancy by everting the cervical lips during speculum examination.

The consistency and appearance of cervical mucus reflect hormonal changes, and have no relevance to the colposcopic detection of early cervical cancer. The cervical mucus undergoes characteristic changes during pregnancy, becoming viscous and cloudy, whitish or yellowish, and containing threads or particles (Figs. 8.**2**, 8.**6**). The mucus can be more difficult to remove with acetic acid than in the nongravid patient.

Are There Pregnancy-Specific Changes?

Apart from lesions such as decidual polyps (Fig. 8.**9**), the colposcopic appearances are not pathognomonic of pregnancy. The same applies to reactive changes, inflammation, and infections.

In the past, there has been lively debate as to whether CIN (SIL) can develop during pregnancy and regress after confinement (2, 9). It is well known that CIN 1–2 (L-SIL) can regress independently of pregnancy. A number of studies, on the other hand, have shown that CIN 3 (H-SIL) detected during pregnancy has not regressed post partum (4, 5, 7, 8). Systematic examination of the cervices of aborting women has even shown a surprisingly high incidence of persisting CIN 3 (5). These results are of interest from the epidemiological point of view and underline the importance of screening during pregnancy.

Effects of Pregnancy on Colposcopic Appearances

Lividity of the cervicovaginal mucosa was one of the clinical signs of pregnancy long before biologic and immunologic tests were developed. This sign is due to the congestion of the pelvic organs, especially the venous plexuses. Marked fluid retention gives the cervix a succulent consistency, and it becomes softer as the pregnancy advances. This development goes hand in hand with the increased lividity. Increased fragility, and a tendency towards contact bleeding, are observed during introduction of the speculum and especially when taking a smear or biopsy (see below).

This lividity and succulence bring about background changes in the colposcopic appearances. In contrast to the nonpregnant state, these are coarse, and may give even benign changes a suspicious and alarming aspect (Figs. 8.**4**–8.**8**). This applies especially to the response to acetic acid.

Acetic Acid Test (p. 20)

The effect of acetic acid is more pronounced during pregnancy, so that whitening even of benign lesions can appear suspicious (Figs. 8.**5**, 8.**6b**, 8.**8b**). The response to acetic acid can thus be difficult to interpret during pregnancy.

The Schiller (Iodine) Test (see p. 23)

The Schiller test is different during pregnancy only to the extent that the cervicovaginal mucosa turns a more intense brownish-black with iodine (Figs. 8.**4b**, 8.**13**, 8.**15b**). The Schiller test is particularly useful when an area that turns white after acetic acid displays a speckled, but not uniform, brown appearance with iodine (Fig. 8.**8c**). Such a finding suggests a condylomatous lesion rather than atypia.

A particularly interesting finding is seen post partum, especially in breast-feeding mothers, when, after a normal colposcopy, several areas on the cervix and vagina do not take up iodine. This epithelium is glycogen-free due to post-partum atrophy (Fig. 8.**21b**). After cessation of breast-feeding, conditions revert to normal, with the usual uniform staining of the vagina and cervix.

Benign Changes in Pregnancy

At the beginning of pregnancy, the cervix can be largely unchanged (Fig. 8.**1**) or display a preexistent condition, such as the coarse grape-like appearance of ectopy. The longitudinal folds of the cervical mucosa are particularly distinctive (Fig. 8.**2**). Such appearances can be caused merely by everting the endocervical canal with the speculum. The coarsening of the surface contour of the transformation zone can occur very early in pregnancy (Fig. 8.**4a**). The Schiller test can bring out other diagnostic features, including islands of mature, glycogen-rich epithelium. The indistinct border between the transformation zone and the surrounding iodine-positive cervix is also suggestive of a benign lesion (Fig. 8.**4b**). After acetic acid is applied, a normal transformation zone often turns more intensely acetowhite than usual, with more prominent gland openings (Figs. 8.**3**, 8.**5**). When transformation is complete, one can see retention cysts and gland openings shining through the lucid epithelium (Fig. 8.**2**).

Clearly delineated areas within a normal transformation zone can appear suspicious, especially when they display an intense reaction to acetic acid (Fig. 8.**6a, b**). In pregnancy, this applies especially to acanthotic epithelium, which can also be clearly demarcated from original squamous epithelium and can show mosaic, or punctation or both (Fig. 8.**7**). In such cases, the small size and regular appearance of the mosaic, or delicate and regular punctation, provide helpful diagnostic hints. In the case of some coarser-looking lesions, and certain combinations of changes, it may be difficult or impossible to make an exact colposcopic diagnosis (Fig. 8.**8a–c**).

The decidual reaction can hardly be seen colposcopically, as it manifests itself in the deeper cervical stroma. Decidual polyps, however, can be easily distinguished from conventional endocervical polyps. The latter often are covered by smooth, pink metaplastic squamous epithelium (Fig. 7.**99**), or display the typical grape-like pattern of columnar epithelium. Decidual polyps, on the other hand, are yellowish, and not covered by epithelium (Figs. 8.**9**, 8.**11**).

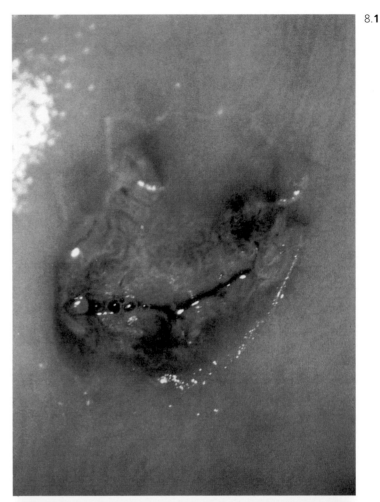

8.**1**

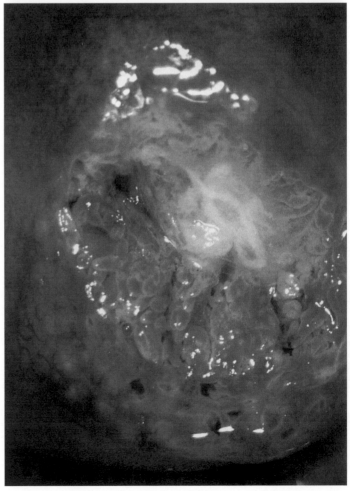

8.**2**

Fig. 8.**1   Gravida 5, 10th week of gestation. Narrow transformation zone** around the external os, slight lividity

Fig. 8.**2   Gravida 3, 17th week of gestation. Ectropion of the cervical mucosa,** with a coarsened texture and deep longitudinal folds. On the posterior lip, the transformation is complete, with gland openings and small cysts shining through. Livid coloration of the entire cervical mucosa. In the os, there is viscous mucus with whitish threads and granules typical of pregnancy

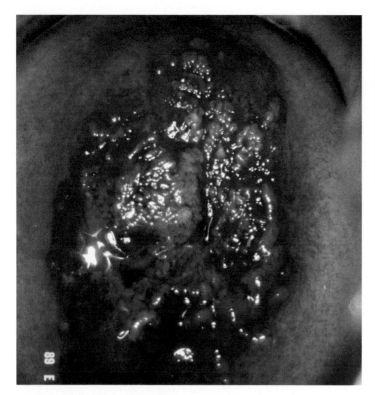

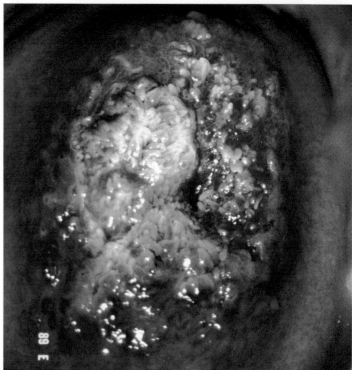

Fig. 8.**3 Gravida 2, 13th week of gestation a** Ectopy and transformation zone with elevated foci of decidual foci on the posterior lip of the cervix

Fig. 8.**3 b** After application of 3% acetic acid, the columnar epithelium swells markedly while the transformation zone and the decidual foci remain largely unchanged

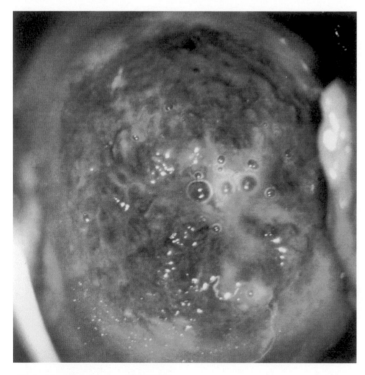

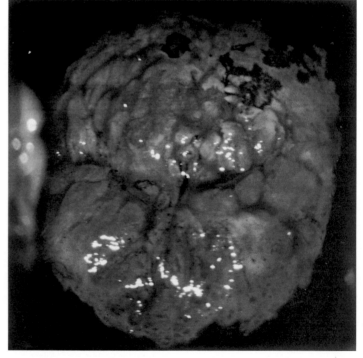

Fig. 8.**4 a Gravida 2, 11th week of gestation. Preexistent transformation zone** with a slightly coarse surface and increased vascularity. Slightly livid coloration of the original cervical epithelium

Fig. 8.**4 b** After the Schiller test, the squamous epithelium is stained dark brown. Within the transformation zone, there are islands of a mature and therefore glycogencontaining metaplastic epithelium

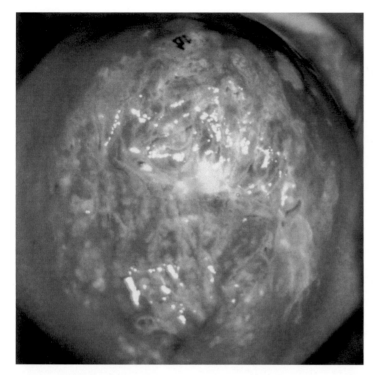

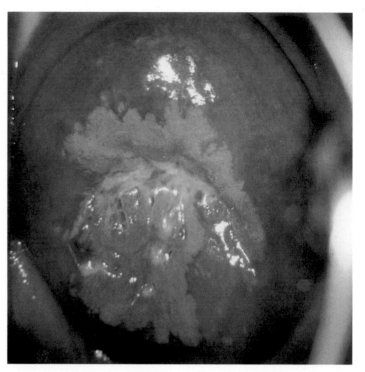

Fig. 8.**5 Gravida 1, 8th week of gestation. Typical transformation zone,** with a whitish reaction to acetic acid. Cuffed gland openings. Flat condylomatous lesions between 12-o'clock and 2-o'clock at the edge of the transformation zone and just outside it

Fig. 8.**7 Gravida 1, 11th week of gestation.** After acetic acid, a white area with fine mosaic and punctation appears on the anterior lip and on the posterior lip outside an ectopy. The border with the slightly livid original epithelium is sharp. Histology showed acanthotic epithelium

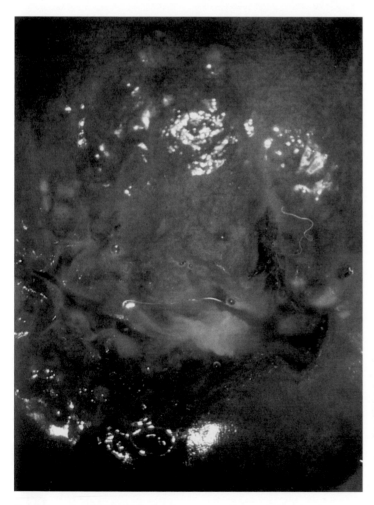

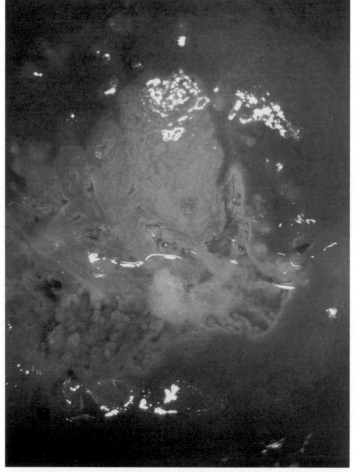

Fig. 8.**6 a Gravida 2, 18th week of gestation.** There is a clearly circumscribed, almost unstructured area within an otherwise unremarkable transformation zone on the anterior lip

Fig. 8.**6 b** A few gland openings and a discrete mosaic appear within the area described after application of acetic acid. Histology showed acanthotic epithelium with mild nuclear irregularities

8.**8a**

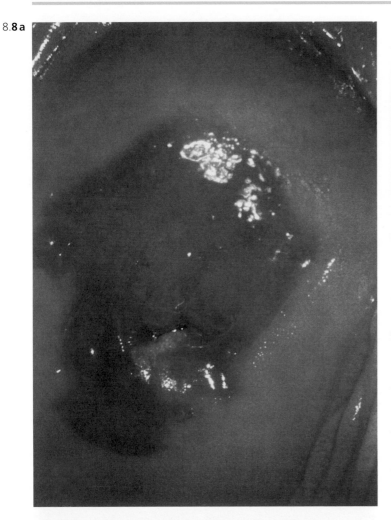

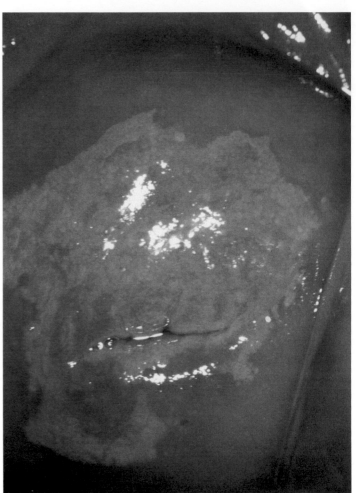

8.**8b**

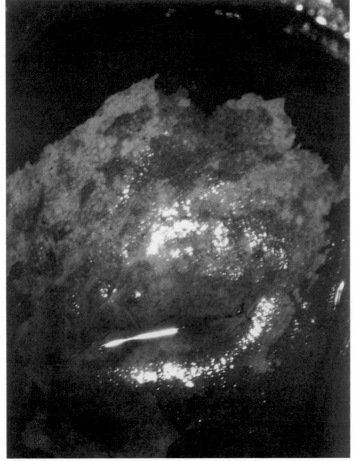

Fig. 8.**8a** **Gravida 1, 11th week of gestation. Shiny red spot** within the livid squamous epithelial covering of the cervix

Fig. 8.**8b** After acetic acid, the entire area turns white, but without swelling. There are small areas of fine mosaic. An isolated field can be delineated between the 11-o'clock and 12-o'clock positions. Histology showed acanthotic epithelium

Fig. 8.**8c** After application of iodine, there is a patchy, partly brown staining of the previously completely white area

Condylomatous lesions are relatively common in pregnancy. Except for a certain succulence, they are similar to those in the nonpregnant patient (Fig. 8.**12**). Inflammatory lesions look the same as they do outside pregnancy. Because the normal epithelium has a deeper brown color, they stand out strongly after iodine (Fig. 8.**13**; see also Fig. 7.**96 b**).

Suspicious Changes

The appearances corresponding to CIN (SIL) are also rather uniform in pregnancy. The distinction between CIN 1 (L-SIL) and acanthotic epithelium is always difficult (Figs. 8.**14**, 8.**6**–8.**8**). However, the irregular, coarser appearance of mosaic, for example, suggests H-SIL in pregnancy as well. The lesions often occur at the periphery of the transformation zone, and in parts also involving the original squamous epithelium (Figs. 8.**15**, 8.**16**). Lividity can give an atypical transformation zone a particular hue (Fig. 8.**17**) that may be overlooked or interpreted as harmless. In other cases, one may find an atypical appearance with intense white coloration of the sharply circumscribed transformation zone (Fig. 8.**18**). Colposcopic le-

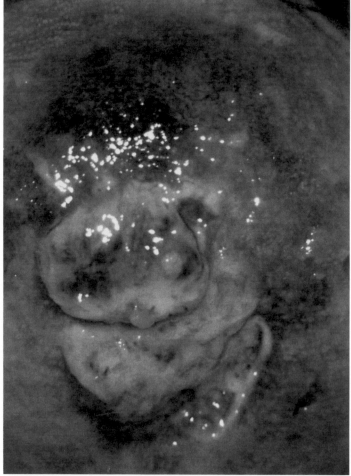

Fig. 8.**9   Gravida 3, 20th week of gestation. Grayish, solid polyps** at the external os. They show no epithelial covering, or any other ▷ superficial structure. Histology showed a decidual reaction

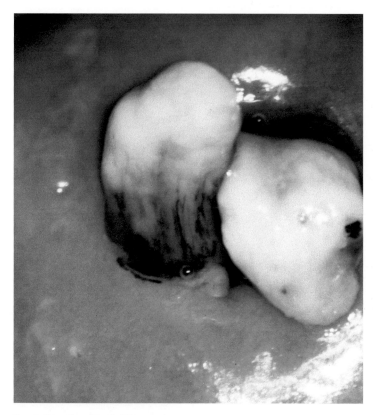

Fig. 8.**10   Gravida 2, 8th week of gestation.** Two decidual polyps in the cervical canal. Their surface is covered with a fibrin which obscures the epithelium. Note the vascular pattern, which is typical for decidual polyps

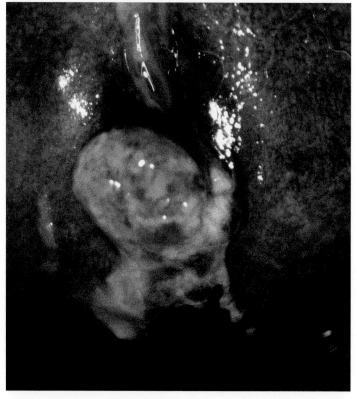

Fig. 8.**11   Gravida 2, 16th week of gestation.** The cervix is livid and there is a decidual polyp in the cervical canal

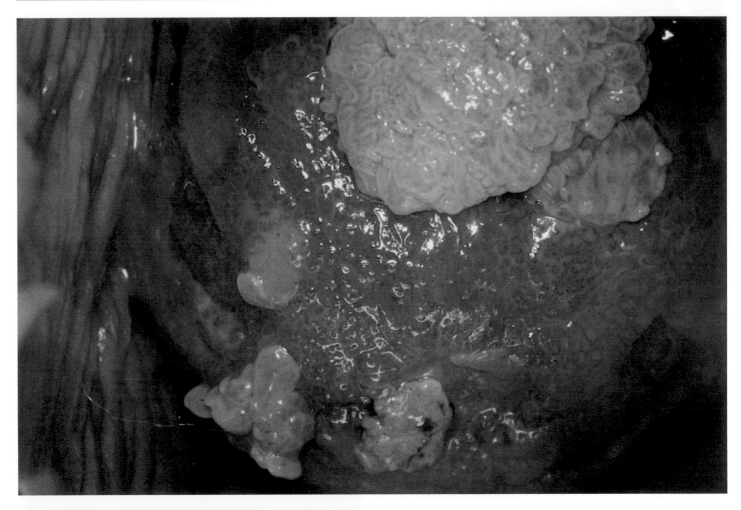

Fig. 8.**12 30th week of gesta-tion.** The vagina and cervix are highly congested. A papillary area around the external os corresponds to flat condylomatous lesions. Within this lesion, and at its edge, there are condylomatous excres-cences which have also assumed a livid red color

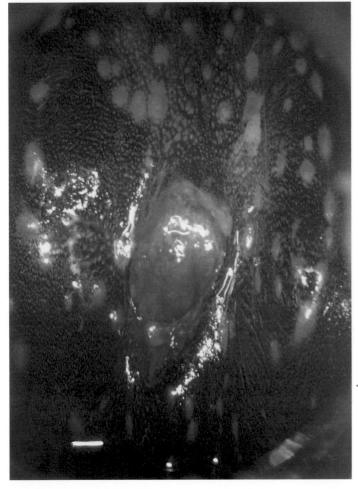

◁ Fig. 8.**13 Gravida 8, 20th week of gestation. Cervix following conization.** The external os is slit-like; the mucosa on the anterior lip is slightly everted. The plaques of a macular colpitis are distinct from the dark brown cervical epithelium

Fig. 8.**14**   **Gravida 1, 20th week of gestation.** Acetic acid has been applied. Outside the transformation zone, on the anterior lip of the external os, there is a fairly fine mosaic, sharply demarcated from its surroundings. Histology showed CIN 1 (L-SIL)   ▷

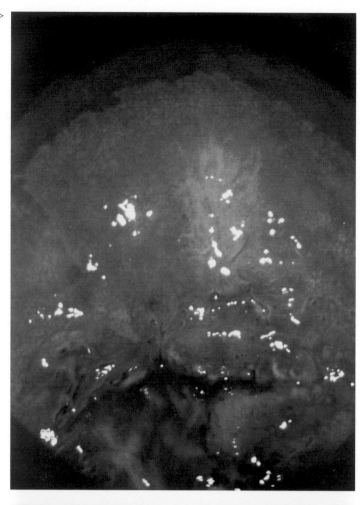

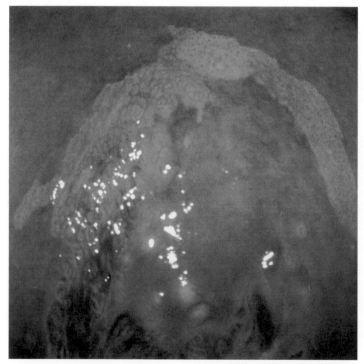

Fig. 8.**15 a**   **Gravida 2. A livid transformation zone** on the anterior lip, with mature epithelium and retention cysts shining through. The transformation zone is semicircularly surrounded by a narrow band of fairly coarse, irregular mosaic. Histology showed CIN 2 (H-SIL)

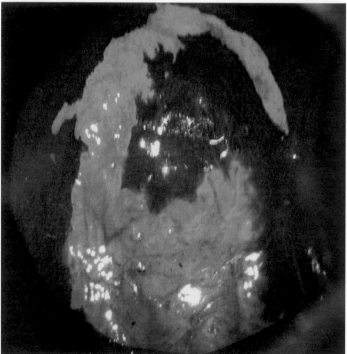

Fig. 8.**15 b**   At a lower magnification, and after the Schiller test, the narrow band with the mosaic is sharply demarcated. The epithelium in the completed transformation zone on the anterior lip is stained dark brown. On the posterior lip, there is an early transformation zone with a diffuse border

8.16

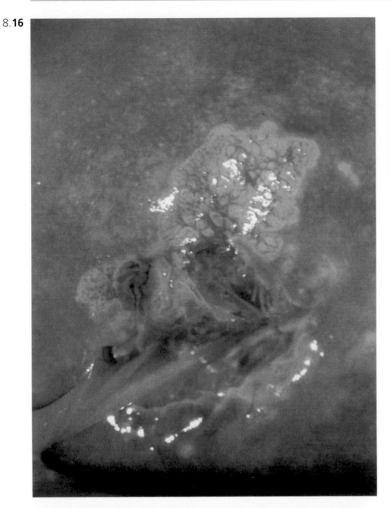

8.17

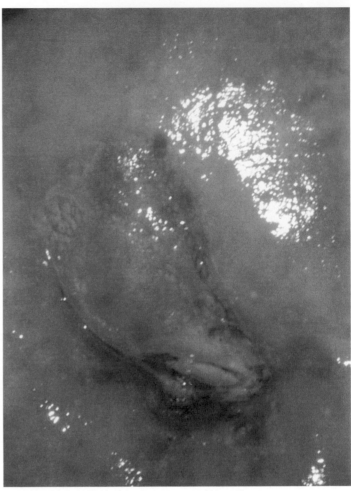

8.18

Fig. 8.**16 Gravida 1, 16th week of gestation.** After application of acetic acid, an irregular, coarse mosaic appears at the edge of, and outside, a small ectopy. Histology showed CIN 2 (H-SIL)

Fig. 8.**17 Gravida 2, 10th week of gestation.** After application of acetic acid, a deeply livid tongue-like area appears on the posterior lip. Within this area, there are only isolated gland openings; at its edge, there is a narrow band with coarse mosaic. Histology showed CIN 2 (H-SIL)

Fig. 8.**18 Gravida 4, 40th week of gestation.** The unusual transformation zone with isolated gland openings is stained intensely white by acetic acid and is sharply demarcated. Histology showed CIN 3 (H-SIL), which was followed closely over the entire pregnancy. The bleeding resulted from a smear taken with a wooden spatula

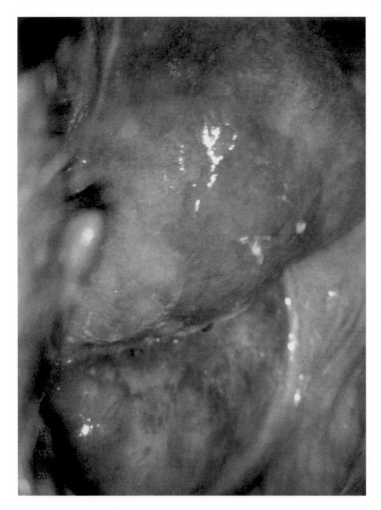

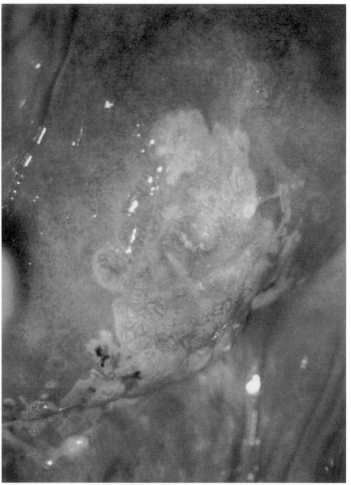

Fig. 8.**19 a Gravida 7, 29th week of gestation.** Within the livid and succulent epithelium, there is a sharply demarcated red area without any recognizable surface structure

Fig. 8.**19 b** After application of acetic acid, the area described swells, and a coarse mosaic appears. Histology showed a carcinoma in situ (CIN 3, H-SIL)

sions, which are bright red and stand out against the livid surroundings, are particularly striking. These are always suspicious, and in cases of H-SIL, also respond characteristically to acetic acid (Fig. 8.**19 a, b**).

Atypical, flat condylomas lose their typical pearly-white appearance (Fig. 7.**91**) during pregnancy. They can even assume a livid undertone, which makes them difficult to recognize as condylomata (Fig. 8.**20 a**). An important diagnostic aid in such cases is the Schiller test, which shows a distinctive brown coloration, with sparing of small clear patches producing a speckled appearance (Fig. 8.**20 b**). This appearance corresponds to the iodine-positive mosaic in Figure 7.**91 b**. If one has an opportunity to observe the lesion during the course of the pregnancy, it can be seen to become coarser, more livid, and more succulent (Fig. 8.**20 c, d**). After confinement, one can observe time and again the regression of condylomatous lesions, leaving a new transformation zone (Fig. 8.**20 e**) which merely displays islands of brown-staining epithelium at the periphery (Fig. 8.**20 f**).

8.20a

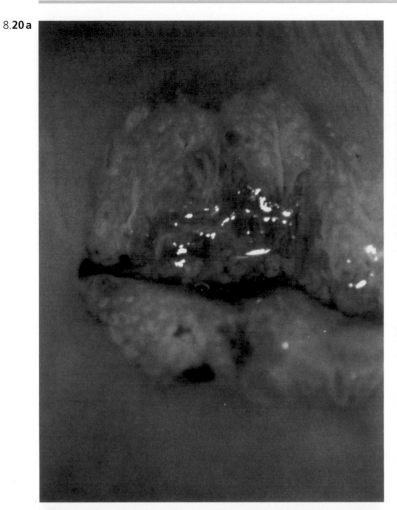

8.20b

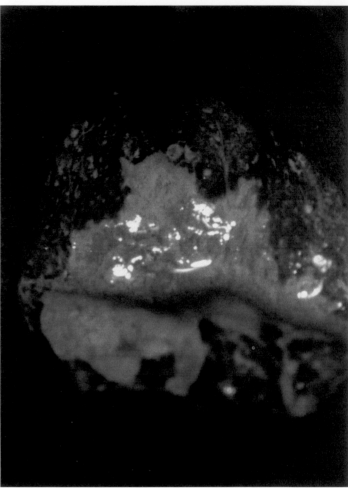

8.20c

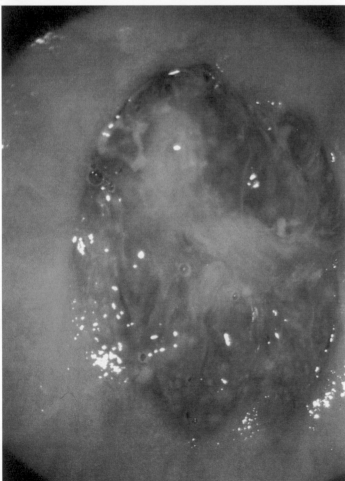

Fig. 8.**20a** **Gravida 2, 8th week of gestation.** At the edge of an ectopy undergoing transformation, there is white-to-livid epithelium with cervical gland openings and white dots. The dots correspond to intraglandular squamous epithelium. Histology showed CIN 2 (H-SIL) with koilocytosis. HPV 16 and HPV 33 positive

Fig. 8.**20b** The brown staining of the epithelium after application of iodine confirms the suspicion of a flat condyloma. The small, light spots could be termed iodine-positive punctation

Fig. 8.**20c** By the 24th week of gestation, the lesion has become coarser and succulent

8.20 d

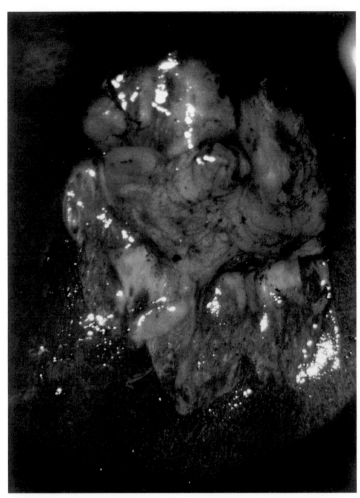

8.20 e

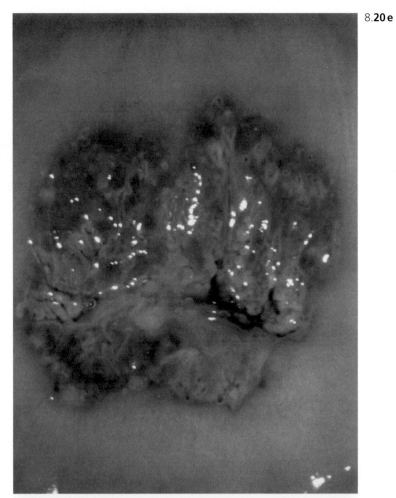

8.20 f

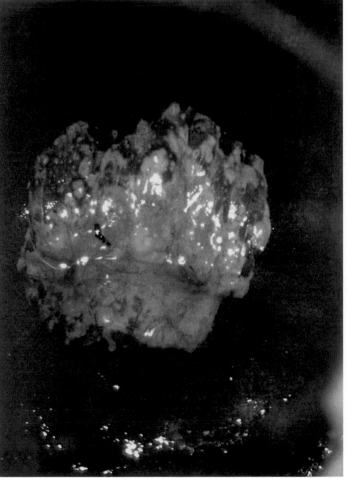

Fig. 8.**20 d** After the Schiller test, the staining of the epithelium on the anterior lip is unchanged. Mucus prevents staining of the posterior lip

Fig. 8.**20 e** Six weeks after delivery, the transformation zone appears normal and bright red. The lesion has become smaller. Histology showed acanthotic epithelium. HPV negative

Fig. 8.**20 f** Application of iodine produces only patchy staining at the edge of the transformation zone

Puerperium

Lesions established during pregnancy remain essentially unchanged during the puerperium; they merely lose the characteristic features imparted by pregnancy (Fig. 8.**20 a–f**). Cases without any changes are often found at the time of the first colposcopic examination after the puerperium (Fig. 8.**21 a**). As mentioned at the outset, it is in such cases that the Schiller test can reveal surprising findings: parts of the cervix and varying lengths of the corrugated surface of the vagina remain unstained, that is, glycogen-free (Fig. 8.**21 b**). This applies especially to breast-feeding women. The appearances completely revert to normal after cessation of lactation. They are probably caused by the hypoestrogenemic state induced by lactation.

Biopsy During Pregnancy

It is quite possible to perform a punch biopsy of the cervix during pregnancy (Fig. 3.**6**). Bleeding can always be controlled with a tampon (Fig. 3.**5**), which should be left in for a few hours. Endocervical curettage can also be performed when indicated; naturally, this should not reach the upper confines of the endocervical canal, where lesions are rare during pregnancy.

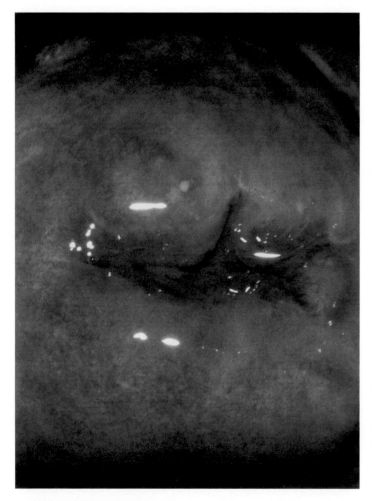

Fig. 8.**21 a**   Four weeks after delivery. The cervix is still slightly red and edematous, with a narrow transformation zone

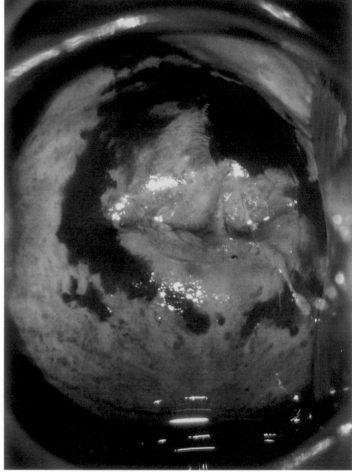

Fig. 8.**21 b**   After the Schiller test, surprisingly large areas of the cervix and vagina are not stained, i.e., glycogen-free. Islands of brown staining appear within these areas

References

1 Coppleson M, Reid B. A colposcopic study of the cervix during pregnancy and the puerperium. J Obstet Gynaecol Br Commonw 1966;73:575.

2 Epperson JWW, Hellman LM, Galvin GA, Busby T. The morphological changes in the cervix during pregnancy, including intraepithelial carcinoma. Am J Obstet Gynecol 1951;61:50.

3 Fluhmann CF. The cervix uteri and its disease. Philadelphia: Saunders, 1961.

4 Green RR, Peckham BM. Preinvasive cancer of the cervix and pregnancy. Am J Obstet Gynecol 1958;75:551.

5 Hamperl K, Kaufmann C, Ober KG. Histologische Untersuchungen an der Cervix schwangerer Frauen. Arch Gynäkol 1954;184:181.

6 Hamperl H, Kaufmann C, Ober KG, Schneppenheim P. Die "Erosion" der Portio. Die Entstehung der Pseudoerosion, das Ektropion und die Plattenepithelüberhäutung der Cervixdrüsen auf der Portiooberfläche. Virchows Arch [A] 1958;331:51.

7 Marsh M, Fitzgerald PJ. Carcinoma in situ of the human uterine cervix in pregnancy. Cancer 1956;9:1195.

8 Moore DB, Gusberg SB. Cancer precursors in pregnancy. Obstet Gynecol 1959;13:530.

9 Nesbitt REL Jr, Hellman LM. The histopathology and cytology of the cervix in pregnancy. Surg Gynecol Obstet 1952;94:10.

10 Stieve H. Der Halsteil der menschlichen Gebärmutter, seine Veränderungen während der Schwangerschaft, der Geburt und des Wochenbettes und ihre Bedeutung. Z Mikroanat Forschung 1927;11:291.

9

Assessment of Colposcopic Findings

Every colposcopist hopes to predict the histology from the colposcopic findings. This is relatively easy as far as original squamous epithelium, ectopy, or completely normal transformation zones are concerned. The task becomes more difficult when the colposcopic findings are abnormal: here the question arises whether the changes are benign or atypical.

These questions become particularly challenging when the colposcopic findings are similar, differing only in subtle features. If these diagnostic features were added to the list of colposcopic findings, the terminology of colposcopy could be expanded and would become the connecting thread for a kind of predictive colposcopy (see p. 40). For this to be useful, the individual criteria allowing a more accurate evaluation of the colposcopic appearances must be well known. But we emphasize that none of these features are pathognomonic of malignancy. They can be expressed to a variable degree, and only facilitate the assessment of colposcopic changes. Any suspicious lesion must be evaluated by cytology and biopsy.

In practice, the colposcopist must distinguish between two patterns: *nonsuspicious findings* and *suspicious findings*.

With experience, the colposcopist will succeed more and more in distinguishing between the two, thereby markedly reducing the number of biopsies. *Suspicious findings* are not synonymous with *abnormal findings* because the latter are not always due to premalignant lesions.

Acanthotic and Atypical Squamous Epithelium

Variations in the interpretation of colposcopic findings are due to the fact that colposcopy is carried out all too often only to evaluate abnormal smears. Patient selection thereby ensures that abnormal colposcopic findings correspond to histologically atypical epithelia in most cases. The few exceptions are so surprising and confusing that they require lengthy and elaborate explanations, rather like an exception to a rule.

Those who use colposcopy routinely take a diametrically opposed view. In their experience the histologic counterparts of leukoplakia, punctation, mosaic or unusual transformation zone are more often acanthotic than atypical epithelia. This has led to the use of the term *malignancy index* (18) in German-speaking countries, which indicates the likelihood of an abnormal colposcopic finding having atypical epithelium as its cause. Table 9.**1** shows the frequency of atypical epithelium or early stromal invasion in biopsies obtained from colposcopically suspicious lesions (1, 18). In cases of leukoplakia, the malignancy index was only 7.4%, while in cases of mosaic and punctation it was 18.6%. Biopsy evaluation of white epithelium (atypical transformation zones) returned a malignancy index of 17% and of colposcopically inconspicuous iodine-negative areas (detected by the Schiller test) of only 1.7%.

Table 9.**1** Malignancy index

Findings at routine colposcopy	CIN (SIL or microinvasion)
Leukoplakia	7%
Mosaic or punctation	19%
Leukoplakia + mosaic + punctation	31%
White epithelium (atypical transformation zone)	17%
Inconspicuous iodine-negative area	2%

(after Bajardi et al. 1959)

The simple explanation for these observations is the so-called *acanthotic epithelium*. European colposcopy has recognized that eight out of ten cases of abnormal colposcopic findings are brought about by acanthotic epithelium (see p. 12). But in English-speaking countries the existence of acanthotic epithelium is not as well-known and is referred to by a bewildering number of terms.

Acanthotic epithelium is a great imitator. Of great significance is the fact that it can arise in the transformation zone. Thus, the metaplastic process can result in completely normal epithelium, atypical epithelium, or acanthotic epithelium. Like the epidermis, it is composed mostly of prickle cells, and shows at least parakeratosis. When arising from original squamous epithelium, it does so from the basal layer (3). It is important for colposcopic diagnosis because acanthotic epithelium can develop in clearly demarcated fields. Normal glycogen-containing epithelium can also change to diffusely keratinizing acanthotic epithelium, as in prolapse (see p. 96).

If the acanthotic epithelium is focal, the individual areas have sharp borders. The surface usually shows parakeratosis or hyperkeratosis. Finally, acanthotic epithelium is very often peg-forming, being subdivided by tall stromal papillae. The pegs can appear as isolated columns or can be arranged in interlacing net-like ridges. Acanthotic epithelium can therefore appear in the transformation zone as leukoplakia, punctation, mosaic, or even acetowhite epithelium.

An appreciation of the significance of acanthotic epithelium is vital to the understanding of colposcopy. Without resorting to complicated explanations and theories, the problem is simply whether an abnormal colposcopic finding is due to disturbed epithelial maturation or to neoplastic epithelial transformation.

Criteria for Differential Diagnosis

A number of features are of value in the differential diagnosis of colposcopic findings:

    a sharp borders,
    b response to acetic acid (white epithelium),
    c surface contour,
    d appearance of gland openings,
    e appearance of blood vessels,
    f surface extent (size),
    g combinations of abnormalities,
    h iodine uptake, and
    i keratinization.

Sharp Borders

Sharp borders are among the most important colposcopic findings. It is amazing how little appreciated this feature is in the colposcopic literature and cervical pathology. The reason for this may be that the existence of pathologic atypia in well-circumscribed fields is not consistent with certain theories of carcinogenesis.

Almost all colposcopically significant lesions have sharp borders. Such borders are also found within large lesions, especially with the Schiller test.

Any sharply circumscribed epithelium must have formed by transformation. Reactive changes, such as those induced by inflammation, are usually diffuse. Sharp borders are often recognizable by native colposcopy. In any case, they become distinct following application of iodine (Fig. 9.**1a**, **b**). In contrast to punctation and mosaic, which are always sharply circumscribed, punctation due to inflammation and mosaic simulated by chance arrangement of blood vessels have indistinct margins. In most cases, the criterion of sharp borders alone enables one to distinguish between significant and nonspecific colposcopic lesions. This feature, however, cannot be used to differentiate between acanthotic and atypical epithelia because both have sharp borders.

Response to Acetic Acid (White Epithelium)

As explained on p. 20, acetic acid clarifies the colposcopic appearance by removing the mucus. Acetic acid also induces swelling of atypical epithelium because of its poor intercellular cohesiveness. At the same time, the epithelium changes from red to white. If, in addition, the lesion displays punctation or mosaic, the white epithelial fields project above the surface. Vascular structures remain red and consequently become better contrasted. The atypical transformation zone remains unstructured except for the gland openings, and thus displays a white surface (Fig. 7.**44**). This feature is called "white epithelium" if neither mosaic nor punctation are present. The cohesiveness of the epithelium is directly proportional to its differentiation, the effect of acetic acid being maximal on undifferentiated epithelium. Thus, its effect on mildly dysplastic epithelium is considerably less than on epithelium showing poorly differentiated carcinoma in situ (Figs. 9.**2**, 9.**3**). Condylomata, especially flat ones, show a characteristic shiny white mother-of-pearl hue (Figs. 7.**89**, 7.**91a**).

9.**1a**

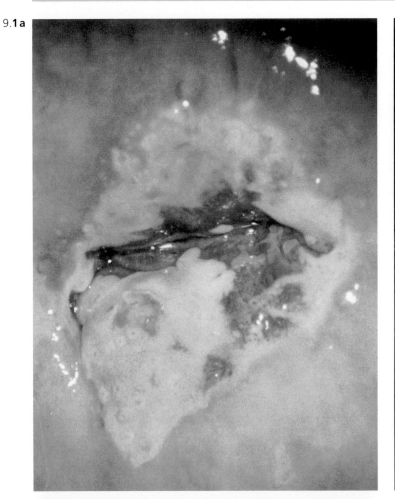

9.**1b**

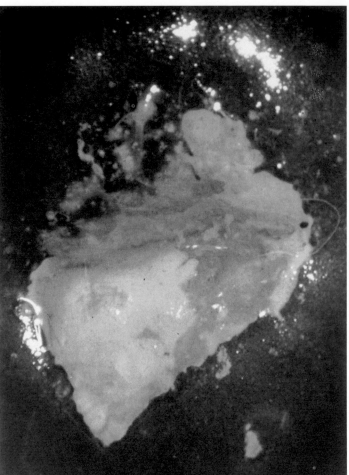

9.**2**

Fig. 9.**1a**   **Atypical transforma-tion zone (white epithelium)** of quite uniform appearance after acetic acid. Note the cuffed gland openings

Fig. 9.**1b**   After application of iodine, it becomes clear that the typically yellowish discoloration is focal and the sharp border segmental. Between the 9-o'clock and 12-o'clock positions, the mar-gin is quite indistinct. The iodine-yellow area returned CIN 3 (H-SIL)

Fig. 9.**2**   **Moderately coarse mosaic** with mild accentuation of the surface contour following ap-plication of acetic acid. Histology showed CIN 2 (H-SIL)

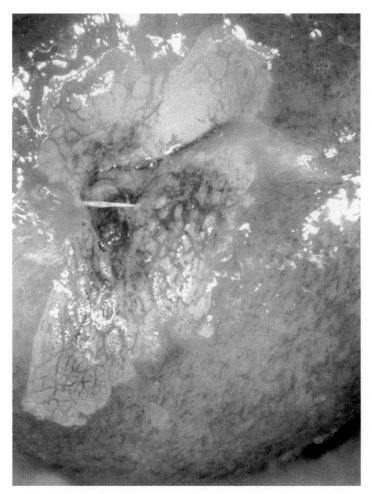

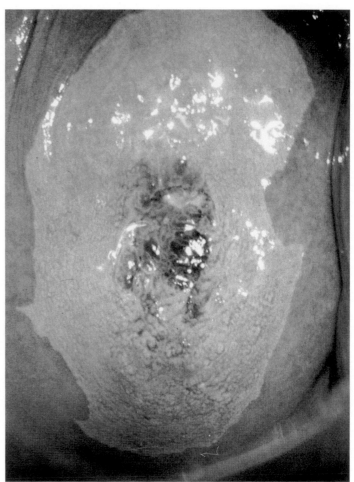

Fig. 9.**3** **Coarse mosaic** with marked swelling and elevation of the epithelium after application of acetic acid. Histology showed carcinoma in situ (CIN 3)

Fig. 9.**4** **Fairly fine mosaic.** The sharply circumscribed acetowhite epithelium remains in the same plane as its surroundings. Histology showed acanthotic epithelium

Surface Contour

Punctation and mosaic produced by acanthotic epithelium resemble a delicate sketch, the dots being small and the lines fine. The distance between the spots is not excessive, and the epithelial fields between the lines are small and regular. All these structures become more distinct following application of acetic acid (Fig. 9.**4**) but do not project from the surface. Punctation produced by atypical epithelium can appear in extreme cases as *elevated papillae* (Fig. 9.**5**) and the lines of mosaic as *coarse ridges* (Fig. 9.**3**). In contrast to acanthotic epithelium, the dots (or papillae) of atypical epithelium are more widely separated; similarly, the epithelial cobbles of a mosaic are larger. These structures become more prominent after application of acetic acid and become raised above the surface. In clear-cut cases, it is easy to differentiate between fine and coarse mosaics and punctations. There is a spectrum of appearances between the two extremes, the proper categorization of which depends on the evaluation of the remaining criteria.

Coarse patterns of punctation and mosaic with an irregular surface configuration can be produced by *flat condylomas* (Fig. 9.**6**), which are essentially benign. Their pearly surface can distinguish them from atypical lesions, the surfaces of which are characteristically matt and opaque. A useful diagnostic feature is the presence of one or more spikes on or near the lesion, as flat condylomas frequently coexist with papillary or spiked condylomas.

Cuffed Gland Openings

The presence of gland openings is a characteristic feature of the transformation zone. They are visible proof that columnar epithelium has been replaced by squamous epithelium. The metaplasia is often restricted to the rims of the gland outlets, leaving the mouths open. The metaplasia can also involve the glandular crypts. In such cases, the gland openings will be completely lined by squamous epithelium. Colposcopically, such events are evidenced by the development of white rings after application of acetic acid (Fig. 7.**14**). If the epithelium is atypical, the ring will be wider and more pronounced after acetic acid (Fig. 7.**44**) than when the epithelium is normal or acanthotic (Figs. 7.**14**, 7.**17**). Such an appearance is referred to as a "cuffed gland opening."

9.**5**

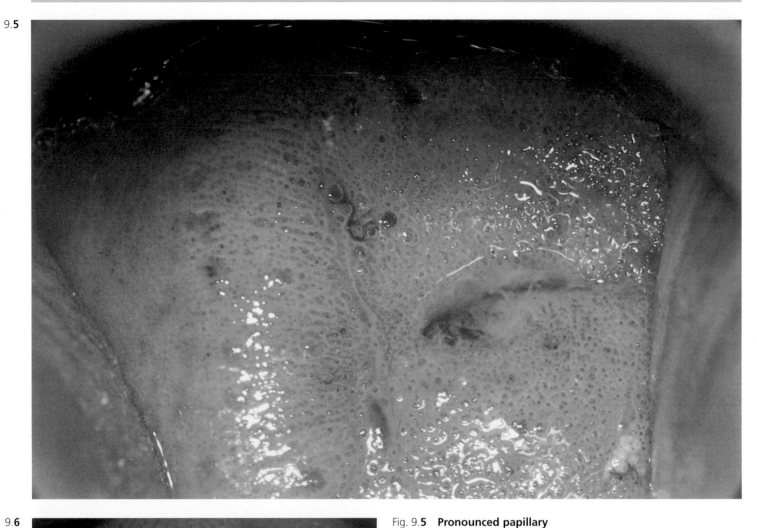

Fig. 9.**5 Pronounced papillary punctation.** Histology showed carcinoma in situ (CIN 3) with early stromal invasion

9.**6**

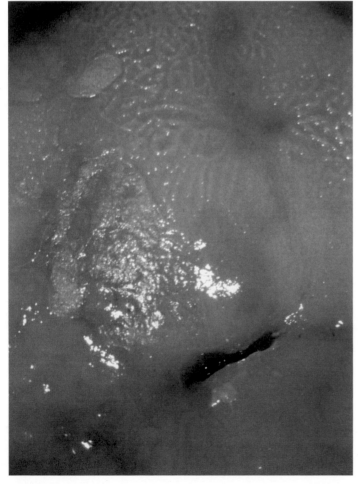

Fig. 9.**6 Flat condylomatous lesions** with gyrated surfaces. In between, there are small, markedly cornified areas (HPV negative)

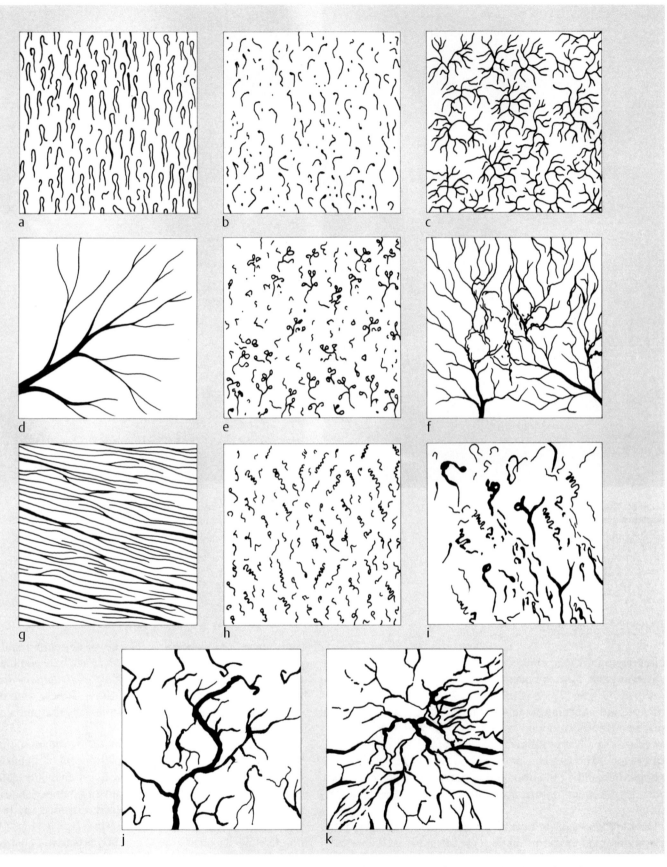

Fig. 9.7 Normal and atypical vascular patterns on the cervix.
a Hairpin-shaped capillary loops.
b Comma-shaped capillaries.
c Blood vessels with regular branching. **d** Long regularly branching vascular tree, with gradual decrease in caliber.
e Staghorn-like vessels, seen especially in inflammation.
f Regular vascular network, simulating mosaic. **g** Long parallel-coursing blood vessels, with some variation in caliber. **h** Irregular corkscrew vessels that vary only slightly in caliber. **i** Bizarre, tortuous, atypical vessels, with marked variation in caliber. **j** Atypical blood vessels with gross variation in caliber and arrangement and abrupt changes in direction.
k Irregular vessels with great fluctuation in caliber

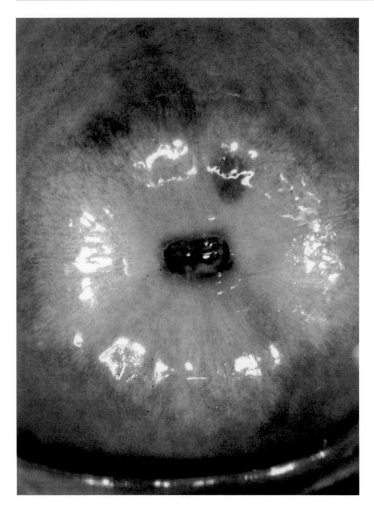

Fig. 9.**8** **Thin, atrophic squamous epithelium** allows the fine radial network of blood vessels to shine through; the vascular pattern is not suspicious (compare with Fig. 9.**12**)

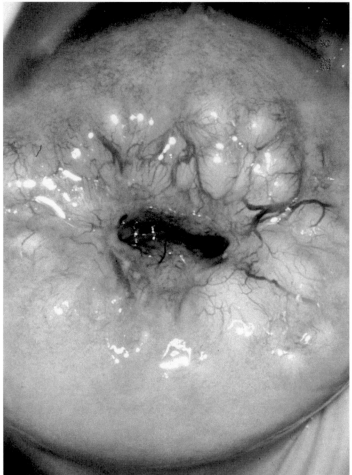

Fig. 9.**9** **Typical vascular tree** of a nabothian follicle; note the regular branching

Blood Vessels

Hinselmann (5, 7) attributed a great deal of importance to the vascular pattern, which became the subject of numerous studies (9, 10, 13, 16, 17, 19, 20). The nature of the blood vessels provides an important diagnostic clue. The vasculature of the thick and well-developed squamous epithelium of reproductive life is not always visible. The same applies to that of an intact ectopy. The vascular pattern, however, is enhanced by inflammation and by the attenuation of the covering epithelium, and is a prominent feature of well-circumscribed epithelial lesions.

The blood vessels are best observed at the beginning of the colposcopic examination. Acetic acid can suppress the vasculature to the point that it almost disappears (see Fig. 7.**31**). Applying a solution of ornipressin (5 IU diluted with 2 ml saline) induces a reactive dilatation and makes the vessels become more prominent (8). A green filter, which screens out red and makes the vessels appear dark, can enhance the vascular appearance. Like other authors (14, 17, 20), we distinguish between various vascular patterns.

Nonsuspicious Vascular Pattern

The course and branching of the vessels are regular, with gradual reduction in caliber. The distance between the regular terminal capillary loops, the so-called *intercapillary distance*, is normal (Fig. 9.**7a–f**). The distribution of these vessels is usually diffuse, and they do not appear in lesions that are clearly circumscribed.

Such vessels are characteristic of diffuse inflammation, when the cervix assumes a stippled appearance. On higher magnification, the capillary loops are hairpin or, when not seen in their entirety, comma-shaped. Diagnostic difficulties can arise if the inflammatory foci are not regularly disposed, as in colpitis macularis, but vary in size and distribution (see Fig. 7.**94**). The blood vessels in such lesions can be particularly clearly etched out and can be fork-shaped or antler-shaped; the intercapillary distance, however, remains normal. The appearances can mimic punctation. These lesions are always poorly circumscribed, a feature seen especially well after application of iodine.

The neat, finely-knit meshwork of blood vessels of atrophic, postmenopausal squamous epithelium can be distinctive (Fig. 9.**8**).

9.**10**

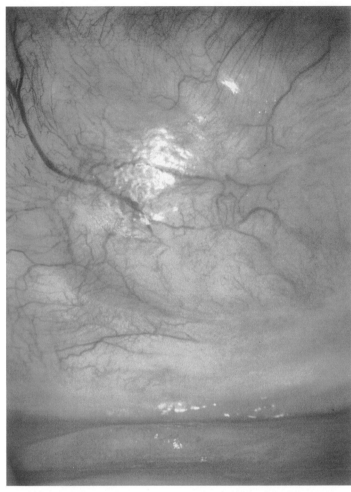

9.**11**

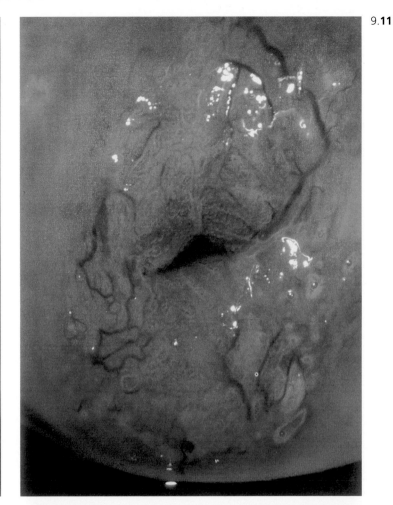

Fig. 9.**10 Long, regularly branching blood vessels** coursing over the surface of a deep nabothian follicle; note the gradual decrease in their caliber

Fig. 9.**11 Atypical transformation zone.** Long vessels with slight variation in caliber and some abrupt changes in direction. Histology showed CIN 1 (L-SIL) with koilocytosis

Fig. 9.**12 Detail of an atypical transformation zone (white epithelium)** with various types of atypical vessels. Histology showed carcinoma in situ (CIN 3, H-SIL)

9.**12**

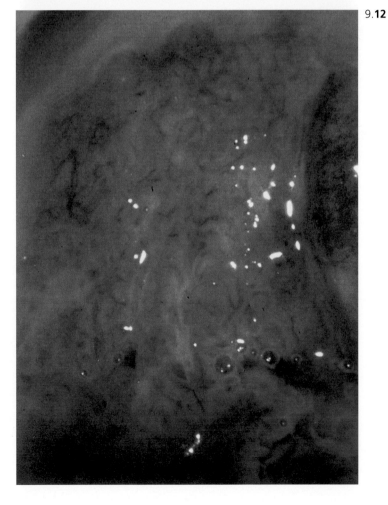

The individual vessels of the vascular network of the normal transformation zone tend to be long and regularly arborizing, with no abrupt change in direction or in caliber. The vessels decrease in caliber as they branch out. Nabothian follicles classically display normal vascular patterns. The long blood vessels that traverse these yellowish structures are relatively large and show regular branching and gradual loss of caliber (Fig. 9.**9**). They are so characteristic that the presence of deep-seated and otherwise invisible nabothian follicles can be deduced (Fig. 9.**10**).

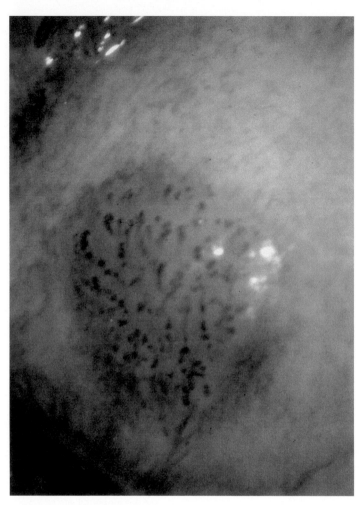

Fig. 9.**13 Coarse, tortuous, comma-shaped and corkscrew-shaped vessels** that vary distinctly in caliber. The intercapillary distance is markedly increased. Histology showed carcinoma in situ (CIN 3) with early stromal invasion

Suspicious Vascular Pattern

The first hint of atypia is the confinement of blood vessels to sharply circumscribed areas (especially with iodine) (Fig. 9.**7g, h**). The blood vessels in punctation are fine to coarse and hairpin, comma, or tortuous (corkscrew) in shape, but still regularly arranged. Within this pattern, the appearances show wide variation. The capillary loops in punctation due to acanthotic epithelium are delicate and regular, with no increase in the intercapillary distance (see Fig. 9.**7**). The tortuous corkscrew and comma-shaped vessels associated with atypical epithelium are coarser, show haphazard branching, and show great variation in caliber; the intercapillary distance is increased (Fig. 9.**11**).

A similar range of appearances is seen in the various expressions of mosaic. The delicate mosaic pattern associated with acanthotic epithelium is produced by small, evenly distributed epithelial fields subdivided by thin red ridges (Fig. 9.**4**). In coarse mosaic, the dividing lines are more definite, the resulting fields larger and more irregular (Fig. 9.**3**).

Even relatively regular and more or less parallel vessels can appear suspicious when they are wider (compare Figs. 9.**8**, 9.**14**) and show an abrupt change in caliber (Fig. 9.**11**).

The vascular pattern can on occasion mimic the appearance of mosaic. Closer inspection, however, will reveal that the vessels in these circumstances display tree-like branching and uniform reduction in caliber, and appear in poorly circumscribed areas (Fig. 9.**7f**).

Atypical Vessels

Atypical vessels show a completely irregular and haphazard disposition, great variation in caliber, and abrupt changes in direction, often forming acute angles (Fig. 9.**7i–k**). The intercapillary distance is increased, and tends to be variable (Fig. 9.**15**).

Highly atypical vessels are characteristic of invasive carcinomas (Figs. 7.**63b**, 9.**16**, 9.**17**), especially when these are clinically overt. When flattish lesions display focal collections of such vessels, microinvasion should be suspected (Fig. 9.**18**).

The 1990 colposcopic terminology includes atypical vessels as a separate diagnostic entity.

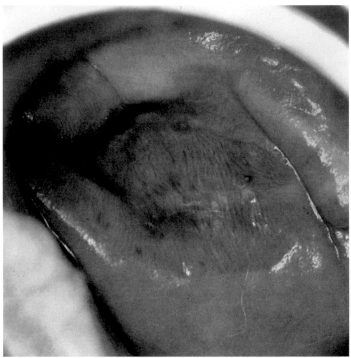

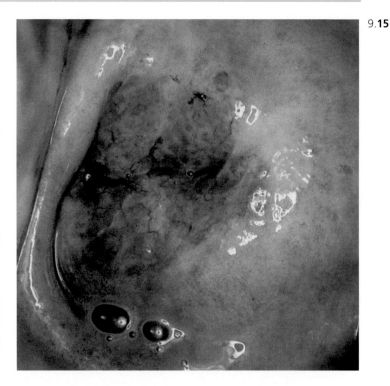

Fig. 9.**14**   **Coarse parallel vessels** showing great variation in caliber, skirting an invasive squamous cell carcinoma

Fig. 9.**15**   **Atypical vessels** showing gross fluctuation in width and abrupt change in direction at the margin of a squamous cell carcinoma within the canal

Fig. 9.**16**   **Highly atypical vessels** on the anterior lip in a partly exophytic and partly endophytic squamous cell carcinoma. Note the complete irregularity and great variation in width

Fig. 9.**17**   **A great variety of atypical vessels** in an invasive squamous cell carcinoma

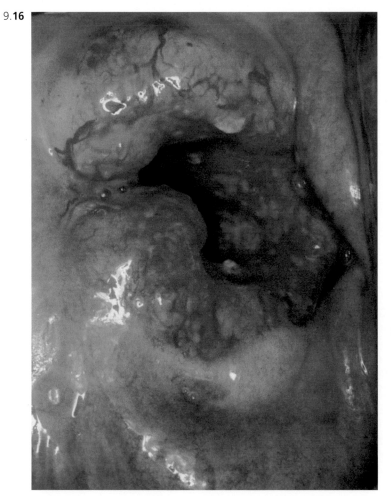

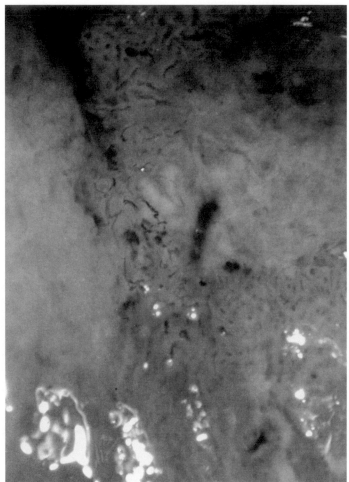

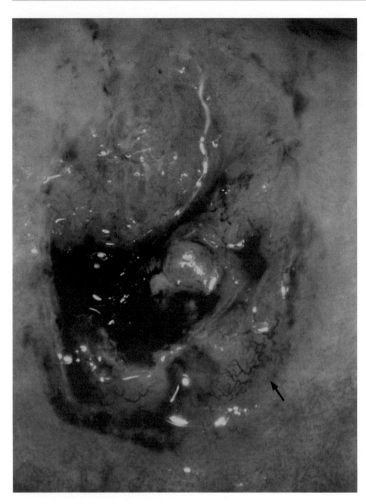

Fig. 9.**18** **Focal collection of atypical vessels** running over the surface of a microcarcinoma on the posterior lip *(arrow)*

Surface Extent (Size)

Morphometric studies of conization specimens have shown that the surface extent of atypical epithelium varies according to its nature, i.e., CIN 1 to 3 (L-SIL to H-SIL) (3, 11). Thus, lesions due to early stromal invasion are larger than those due to carcinoma in situ, which in turn are larger than those due to CIN 2. The same applies even to the various grades of CIN (SIL). This does not mean that fields of carcinoma in situ are larger than those of CIN (SIL) per se, but that the former are more likely to be combined with the latter, the total area thus being larger. The marked increase in the surface extent of early invasive lesions is also due to coalescence of fields of CIN (SIL) and fields of in situ carcinoma (Table 9.**2**). Table 9.**3** shows that the same is true for both cervical lips. There is a direct relationship between size and likelihood of invasion.

The same conclusions apply to colposcopic lesions. Colposcopically suspicious but small lesions are rarely of histologic significance. Conversely, colposcopically highly suspicious lesions are always extensive. Small lesions are much more likely to be CIN (SIL) than in situ or invasive carcinoma. This does not contradict the principles of evaluation of intraepithelial lesions. On the contrary, the coexistence of different epithelia shows that invasive potential is acquired by their coalescence and not by progression of one type to another.

These statements do not apply to acanthotic epithelium, which can involve only small areas or cover the whole cervix and even parts of the vagina.

Consequently, size alone is not a diagnostic criterion; size should be considered only in concert with other criteria. If the latter point to atypia, large size should further raise the index of suspicion.

Table 9.**2** Percentage of different types of atypical epithelia within a colposcopic lesion (n = 703)

Maximal diagnosis	CIN 1 (L-SIL) only	All grades of CIN (SIL)	CIN 2 only	CIN 1 and CIN 3	CIN 2 and CIN 3	All grades of CIN and C.I.S.	C.I.S. only
CIN 1 (L-SIL) (n = 60)	100%	0	0	0	0	0	0
CIN 2 (H-SIL) (n = 108)	0	82%	18%	0	0	0	0
CIN 3 (carcinoma in situ, H-SIL) (n = 489)	0	0	0	8%	35%	41%	16%
Early stromal invasion (n = 46)	0	2%	0	0	50%	20%	28%

C.I.S. = carcinoma in situ

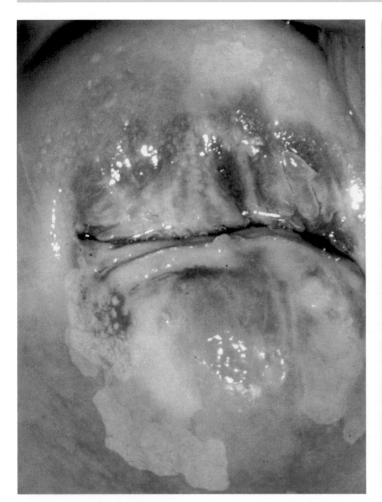

Fig. 9.**19 a** **Acetic acid reveals a raised lesion with a variegated appearance** between 6-o'clock and 8-o'clock. Note the moderately coarse mosaic between 8-o'clock and 9-o'clock

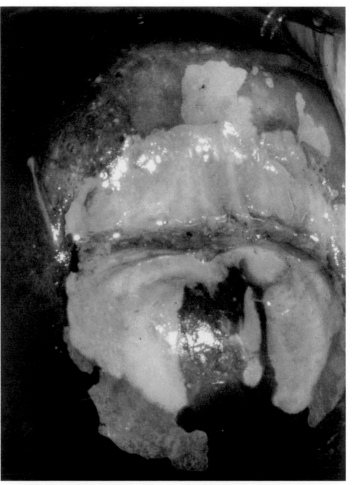

Fig. 9.**19 b** Iodine staining allows a more detailed analysis of an already complex colposcopic picture. The area referred to in Fig. 9.**19 a**, now brownish, is probably a flat condyloma. The brown area on the posterior lip represents fully mature transformed epithelium. The equally well demarcated iodine-yellow area at 12-o'clock is due to acanthotic epithelium. The remaining yellow patches are CIN 3 (H-SIL)

Table 9.**3**   Surface extent of atypical epithelium on the lips of the cervix

	Cases	One lip		Both lips	
CIN 1 (L-SIL)	27	21	(78%)	6	(22%)
CIN 2 (H-SIL)	30	17	(57%)	13	(43%)
Carcinoma in situ (CIN 3, H-SIL)	87	36	(41%)	51	(59%)
Early stromal invasion	66	10	(15%)	56	(85%)

Combinations of Abnormalities

Table 9.**1** (p. 116) lists the *malignancy index* of the various suspicious colposcopic findings. No single lesion exceeds the 20% mark. But if the patterns of leukoplakia, mosaic, and punctation are combined, the chance of finding histologically atypical epithelium climbs to 31%. These facts are entirely consistent with the observation that significant lesions are a patchwork of several epithelial types, including those showing various degrees of atypia (see Figs. 10.**1**–10.**4**).

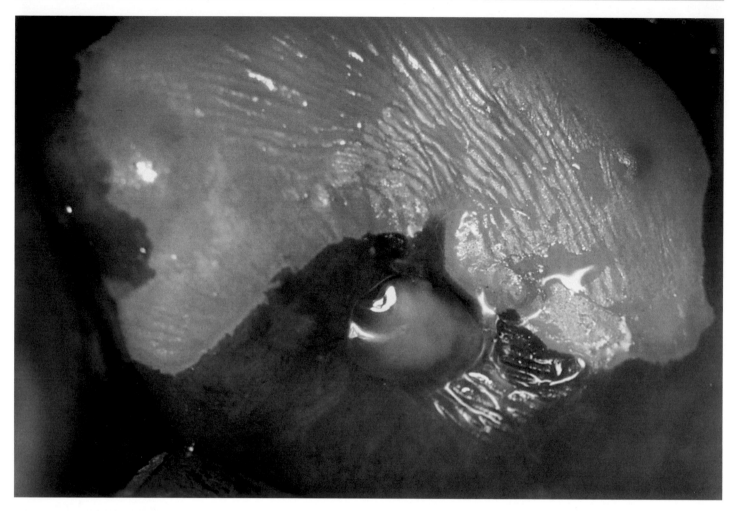

Fig. 9.**20** **Sharply circumscribed,
smooth, iodine-yellow lesion**
due to acanthotic epithelium

Iodine Uptake

Quite apart from enhancing the abruptness of epithelial borders, the staining of colposcopic lesions with iodine is variegated (see also p. 23). Brownish or brown staining due to glycogen should diminish one's suspicions (Fig. 9.**19 a, b**). An area that does not take up iodine at all can be due to columnar epithelium or thin, regenerating, nonspecific epithelium (see Figs. 4.**6** and 4.**7**). Well-developed acanthotic epithelium characteristically stains uniformly canary-yellow, and remains flat (Fig. 9.**20**). Atypical epithelium also stains canary-yellow, but it becomes mottled, and its surface is not so smooth. In cases of punctation and mosaic, the surface contour remains more clearly visible when the epithelium is atypical and not acanthotic, as the latter is essentially flat; the same applies when the Schiller test is used.

Keratinization

Keratinization is not a particularly useful diagnostic criterion. All grades of keratinization, from mild parakeratosis to pronounced hyperkeratosis, can be shared by acanthotic and atypical epithelia, both of which appear colposcopically as leukoplakia. However, a mild degree of keratinization often corresponds to acanthotic epithelium, while flaky keratin suggests epithelial atypia.

The keratin layer obscures not only the surface contour but eventually also the margins, and inhibits the effect of acetic acid. There is poor uptake of iodine, resulting in a light yellow color. If the keratin layer can be peeled off, features of diagnostic importance may emerge. All cases of leukoplakia should be evaluated by biopsy or at least by repeated cytology.

Evaluation of the Differential Diagnostic Criteria

The diagnostic features described above can be expressed to varying degrees, and can be found singly or in combination. *The more distinct a feature is and the greater the variety of features seen in combination, the higher the index of suspicion.* All lesions must be viewed with a high degree of suspicion by the beginner, who should evaluate his or her findings by biopsy as part of the learning process. Quality can also be improved by repeating the smear if this was initially negative. With increasing practice, the colposcopist will be able to distinguish between *benign* and *suspicious findings* with some confidence.

Attempting to differentiate between the various grades of CIN (SIL) colposcopically is more questionable, as these lesions are regarded now as forming a spectrum of the same biologic process (see p. 10).

References

1 Bajardi F, Burghardt E, Kern H, Kroemer H. Nouveaux résultats de la cytologie et de la colposcopie systématiques dans le diagnostique précoce du cancer du col del'utérus. Gynécol Prat 1959;5:315.

2 Burghardt E. Über die atypische Umwandlungszone. Geburtshilfe Frauenheilkd 1959;19:676.

3 Burghardt E. Early histological diagnosis of cervical cancer. Philadelphia: Saunders, 1973.

4 Burke L, Antonioli D, Rosen S. Vaginal and cervical squamous cell dysplasia in women exposed to diethylstilbestrol in utero. Am J Obstet Gynecol 1978;132:437.

5 Hinselmann H. Die Ätiologie, Symptomatologie und Diagnostik des Uteruscarcinoms. In: Veit J, Stöckel W, eds. Handbuch der Gynäkologie, vol. 6.1. Munich: Bergmann, 1930:854.

6 Hinselmann H. Einführung in die Kolposkopie. Hamburg: Hartung, 1933.

7 Hinselmann H. Der Nachweis der aktiven Ausgestaltung der Gefäße beim jungen Portiokarzinom als neues differentialdiagnostisches Hilfsmittel: Zentralbl Gynäkol 1940;64:1810.

8 Horcajo M. Über den Wert der Anwendung eines vasokonstriktorischen Peptids als Zusatzuntersuchung der Kolposkopie. Geburtshilfe Frauenheilkd 1976;36:388.

9 Ganse R. Atypische Gefäßentwicklung beim Portiokarzinom. Zentralbl Gynäkol 1952;74:749.

10 Ganse R. Die atypische Gefäßneubildung bei Karzinom. Zentralbl Gynäkol 1957;79:519.

11 Holzer E., H. Pickel Die Ausdehnung des atypischen Plattenepithels der Zervix. Arch Geschwulstforschung 1975;45:79.

12 Kishi Y, Inui S, Sakamoto Y. Colposcopic findings of gland openings in cervical carcinoma: their histological backgrounds. Int J Gynecol Obstet 1987;25:223.

13 Koller O. The vascular pattern of the uterine cervix. Oslo: Universitetsforlaget, 1963.

14 Kolstad P., Stafl A. Atlas of colposcopy. Oslo: Universitetsforlaget, 1982.

15 Madej J. Significance of vascular changes in the colposcopic diagnosis of precancerous and early stages of cervical cancer. Geburtshilfe Frauenheilkd 1983;43:606.

16 Marsh M. Original site of cervical carcinoma: topographical relationship of carcinoma of the cervix to the external os and to the squamocolumnar junction. Obstet Gynecol 1956;7:444.

17 Mateu-Aragonés JM. Atlas de colposcopia. Barcelona: JIMS, 1973.

18 Navratil E. Colposcopy. In: Gray LA, ed. Dysplasia, carcinoma in situ and microinvasive carcinoma of the cervix uteri. Springfield, IL: Thomas, 1964.

19 Rieper JP, Marcones-Fonseca N. Patologia cervical. São Paolo: Manole, 1978.

20 Zinser HK, Rosenbauer KA. Untersuchungen über die Angioarchitektonik der normalen und pathologisch veränderten Cervix uteri. Arch Gynäkol 1960;194:73.

10

Colposcopic-Histologic Correlation

Ideally, the purpose of colposcopy is to correlate colposcopic findings with the underlying histology. Each colposcopic finding should have an exact histologic counterpart. But such correlations can never be achieved fully, and should not be attempted during routine colposcopy. In daily practice the goal is to distinguish between normal and suspicious findings.

Precise correlations between colposcopic and histologic findings require guided biopsies (1). But analyzing complex colposcopic findings by innumerable biopsies is neither feasible nor fair to the patient. Colposcopic-histologic correlations require good colpophotographs and meticulous histology of conization specimens with serial sections. We have carried out numerous such studies. Many of the legends to the colpophotographs in this book highlight details revealed by comparing colposcopic and histologic findings in conization specimens. To illustrate the kind of information that can be obtained by this kind of analysis, this chapter shows cases that contain multiple abnormal findings. A few of the figures in this chapter also show changes outside the transformation zone, that is outside the glandular field. The heavily dotted lines in the figures mark the borders of the gland field, i.e., the position of the last gland.

Borders within colposcopic lesions are not always easy to recognize, particularly in photographs. Nevertheless, borders become surprisingly distinct with careful scrutiny and with sketching from colpophotographs. Perusal of the photographs will confirm the variety of findings.

First, it becomes obvious that all uniform epithelia arise in clearly circumscribed fields. Second, more differentiated lesions are found distal (toward the vagina) to less-differentiated lesions. Thus, carcinoma in situ (CIN 3, H-SIL) lies above (i.e., further toward or in the cervical canal) than CIN 1 (L-SIL) and 2. Acanthotic epithelium is located most distally (Figs. 10.**1**–10.**3**). All kinds of epithelia are found within the last gland, but they follow these rules (Figs. 10.**1**–10.**4**). CIN 1 and CIN 2 (L-SIL) are found on either side of the last gland, and often begin or end here. Thus, colposcopy illustrates the importance of the histologic concept of the last gland.

To complete the picture, Figure 10.**3** shows the rare exception. There is a large area of CIN (SIL) on both sides of the last gland on the posterior lip of the cervical os. The lesion is uniform and continuous. If the corresponding colpophotograph is studied carefully, the somewhat coarse mosaic is seen to consist of two clearly distinct fields. In this case the two epithelia, which can hardly be distinguished from one another histologically, have arisen quite independently on either side of the last gland. The border of the glandular field at 2 o'clock is covered by normal squamous epithelium that must have arisen in the glandular field by metaplasia.

Figure 10.**4** is instructive because it shows clearly a focus of invasive carcinoma without striking diagnostic features.

Cervical cancer has often been thought to arise only in the transformation zone. Convincing histologic evidence that CIN (SIL) can arise outside the transformation zone, in the original squamous epithelium, has been met with skepticism by colposcopists contending that colposcopic lesions appear uniform. But their view ignores the fact that even uniform lesions can occur simultaneously both inside and outside the glandular field. Although the combination of different colposcopic findings is well known, it is little appreciated that their sharp borders can be seen colposcopically. Naturally, there are lesions that arise completely outside the transformation zone, some exclusively from original squamous epithelium (Figs. 7.**25**, 7.**26a, b**, 7.**33**, 7.**36**, 7.**52**). Even these findings are dismissed by those who maintain that glands must have existed there before. Yet an ectopic cervical mucosa will usually be replaced via metaplasia by squamous epithelium. But the glands beneath the new squamous epithelium remain, as is the case in so-called "occult (vaginal) adenosis" (5). For the same reason, the argument that the last gland is not really the last because others have disappeared, is not valid. If this were so, the position of the last gland would have to be random. The unique topographic relationship of the last gland to epithelial abnormalities, both histologically and colposcopically (Figs. 10.**1**, 10.**4**) is incontestable proof of the validity of the concept of the last gland (2–5).

The Topography of Abnormal Colposcopy Findings

The colposcopic terminology formulated by the International Federation for Cervical Pathology and Colposcopy (IFCPC) in 1990 takes into account that abnormal colposcopy findings can be located inside or outside the transformation zone, or both (15).

The first colposcopic findings, described by Hinselmann, were mosaic, punctation, and leukoplakia (10). Later, Glatthaar (9) and Hinselmann himself recognized lesions in the transformation zone that did not fit Hinselmann's classic matrix areas. These are the lesions now called acetowhite epithelium (even though mosaics and punctations that have developed via atypical epithelium can be markedly acetowhite).

We have studied the frequency with which colposcopically visible lesions were limited to or outside of the histologic transformation zone by correlating colpophotographs with histologic mapping based on step-serial sections of 118 conization specimens (13). The cervical gland field and its borders were reconstructed and epithelial lesions were related to histologic landmarks to reconstruct the topography of the entire cervical epithelium (Fig. 10.**5**). Acetowhite epithelium (Fig. 10.**6**), which develops via atypical squamous metaplasia, accounted for almost half the lesions (Fig. 10.**7**). Thirty-one epithelial lesions were located exclusively within the transformation zone (Table 10.**1**) (Fig. 10.**8**), and two lesions were located exclusively outside the transformation zone (Table 10.**2**) (Fig. 10.**9**). Eighty-five specimens showed abnormal colposcopy findings both within and outside the transformation zone. Of lesions outside the transformation zone, 21 specimens contained two and 10 contained three different lesions simultaneously (Table 10.**3**). The histologic correlates of the mosaics and punctations are shown in Figure 10.**10**. The colposcopic findings within the transformation zone in these 85 patients are summarized in Table 10.**4**. Forty-seven specimens contained two and 11 contained three different lesions. Table 10.**5** shows all mosaics and punctations located within the transformation zone and Figure 10.**11** the histologic correlates. Colposcopy showed glands underneath 11 of 18 mosaics and 2 of 7 punctations. Histology showed cervical glands underneath the epithelial lesions in all

(text continues on p. 139)

a

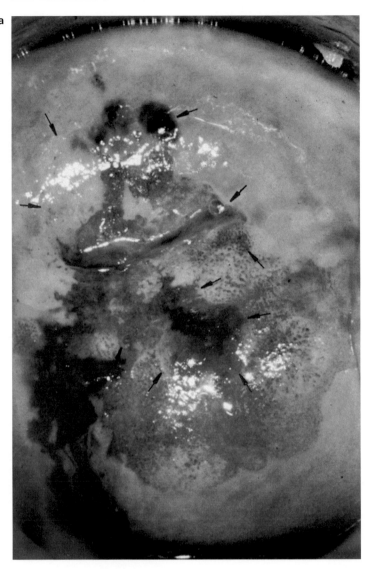

b

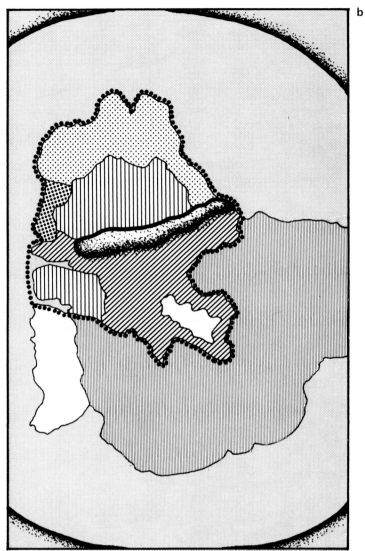

Fig. 10.**1 a, b** **Correlation of the**
colposcopic picture with the
histologic findings in serial step
sections of the corresponding conization specimen. The arrows point
to borders between colposcopic lesions

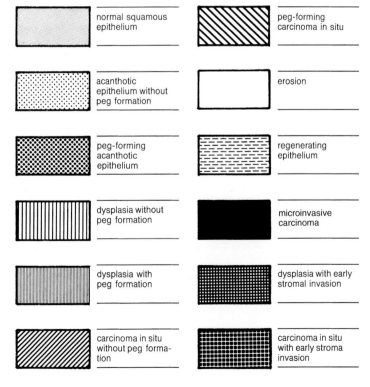

normal squamous
epithelium

peg-forming
carcinoma in situ

acanthotic
epithelium without
peg formation

erosion

peg-forming
acanthotic
epithelium

regenerating
epithelium

dysplasia without
peg formation

microinvasive
carcinoma

dysplasia with
peg formation

dysplasia with early
stromal invasion

carcinoma in situ
without peg forma-
tion

carcinoma in situ
with early stroma
invasion

●●●●●●●●●●●●●●● border of the glandular field

a

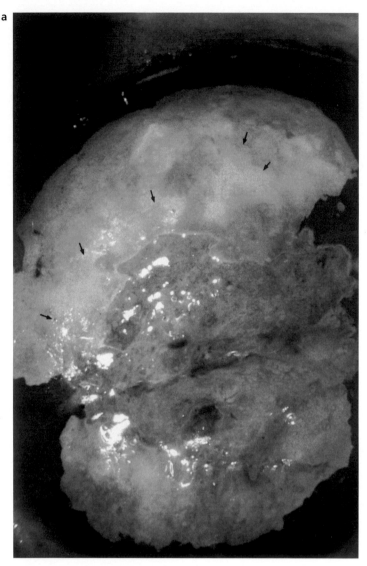

b

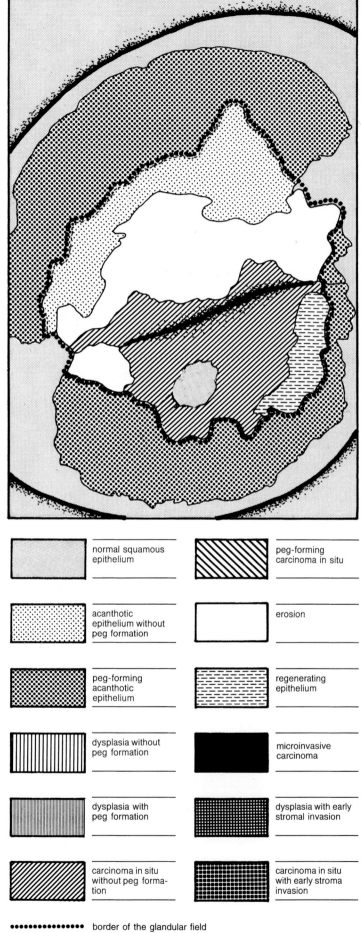

Fig. 10.**2 a, b Correlation of the colposcopic picture following the Schiller test with the histologic findings** in serial step sections of the corresponding conization specimen. The arrows point to discrete borders between colposcopic lesions

normal squamous epithelium

peg-forming carcinoma in situ

acanthotic epithelium without peg formation

erosion

peg-forming acanthotic epithelium

regenerating epithelium

dysplasia without peg formation

microinvasive carcinoma

dysplasia with peg formation

dysplasia with early stromal invasion

carcinoma in situ without peg formation

carcinoma in situ with early stroma invasion

•••••••••••••••• border of the glandular field

a

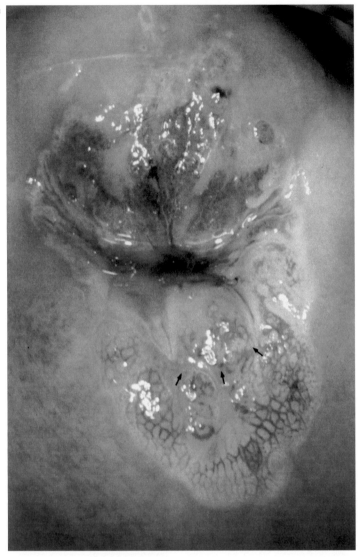

b

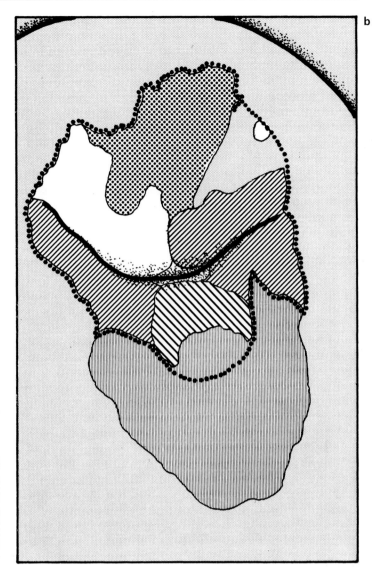

Fig. 10.**3 a, b Correlation of the colposcopic picture with the histologic findings** in serial step sections of the corresponding conization specimen. The arrows point to discrete borders between colposcopic lesions. There is dysplasia on both sides of the last gland

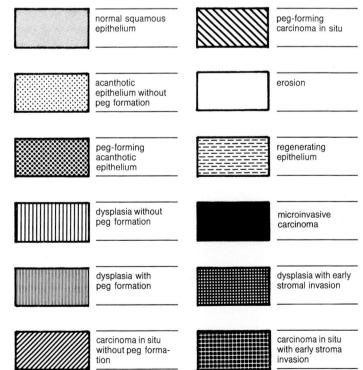

normal squamous epithelium	peg-forming carcinoma in situ
acanthotic epithelium without peg formation	erosion
peg-forming acanthotic epithelium	regenerating epithelium
dysplasia without peg formation	microinvasive carcinoma
dysplasia with peg formation	dysplasia with early stromal invasion
carcinoma in situ without peg formation	carcinoma in situ with early stroma invasion

●●●●●●●●●●●●●●● border of the glandular field

a

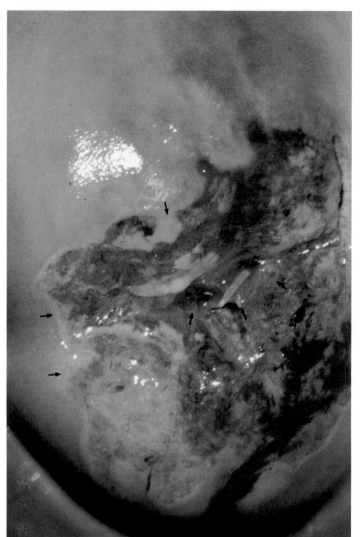

b

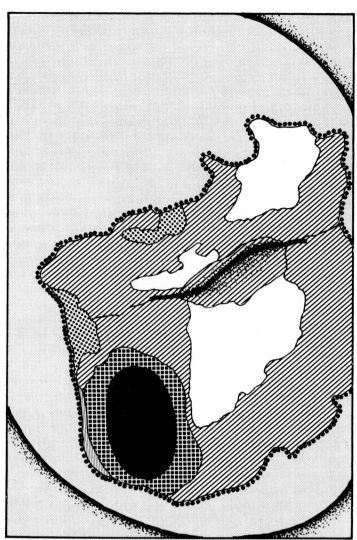

Fig. 10.**4a, b Correlation of the colposcopic picture with the histologic findings** in serial step sections of the corresponding conization specimen. The arrows point to discrete borders between colposcopic lesions

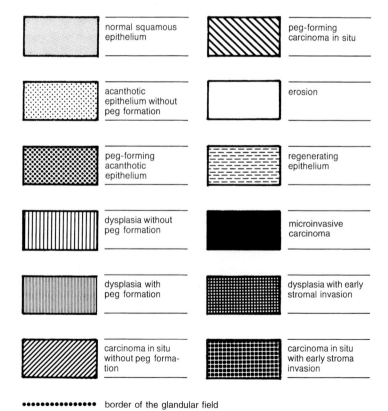

	normal squamous epithelium		peg-forming carcinoma in situ
	acanthotic epithelium without peg formation		erosion
	peg-forming acanthotic epithelium		regenerating epithelium
	dysplasia without peg formation		microinvasive carcinoma
	dysplasia with peg formation		dysplasia with early stromal invasion
	carcinoma in situ without peg formation		carcinoma in situ with early stroma invasion

•••••••••••••••• border of the glandular field

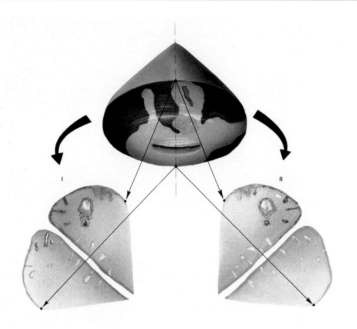

Fig. 10.**5b**

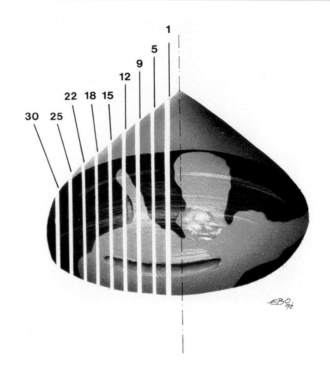

Fig. 10.**5** Schematic representation of the histologic processing of a conization specimen. The cone is divided in half in the sagittal plane (**a**) and processed as step-serial sections at 400-μm intervals (**b**, 1–30). The gland field is reconstructed by connecting the positions of the last glands (**c**, 1–25). The epithelial lesions and the borders between them are then related to the colposcopic findings

Fig. 10.**5c**

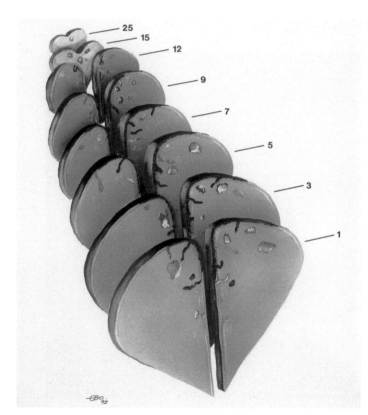

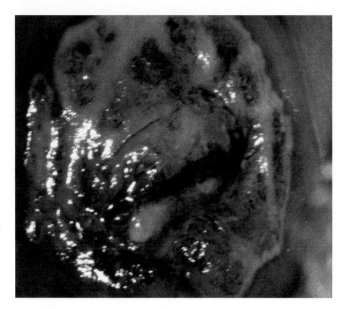

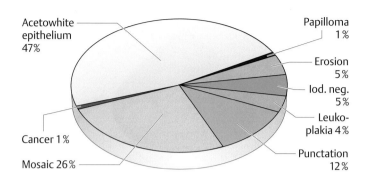

Fig. 10.**7** Distribution of abnormal colposcopy findings in 118 conization specimens

Fig. 10.**6** Acetowhite epithelium. Histology showed CIN 3 (H-SIL)

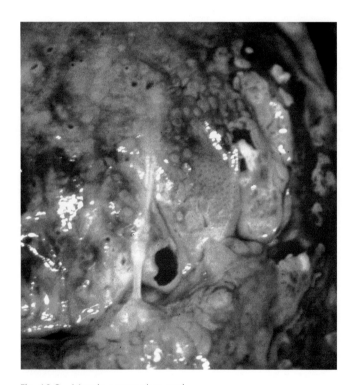

Fig. 10.**8** Mosaic, punctation, and acetowhite epithelium within the transformation zone; histology showed CIN 3 (H-SIL)

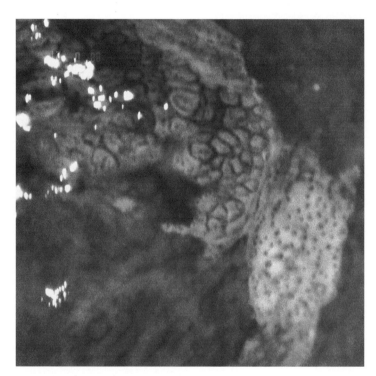

Fig. 10.**9** Mosaic and punctation entirely outside the transformation zone; histology showed CIN 2 (H-SIL)

specimens. Figures 10.**12** and 10.**13** show the histologic correlates of the colposcopic findings iodine-negative area, leukoplakia, and acetowhite epithelium. In 84% of the specimens, the mosaics, punctations, leukoplakias, and colposcopically mute iodine-negative areas were outside the transformation zone—i.e., in the area of the original squamous epithelium; in 16% they were inside the transformation zone.

These results suggest that the classic colposcopic findings of mosaic, punctation, and leukoplakia are primarily lesions of the original squamous epithelium and probably of viral origin. Only acetowhite epithelium develops mainly via squamous epithelial metaplasia (16). This is in contrast to theories that all lesions develop via squamous epithelial metaplasia (7, 13, 14). Also, the histologic results indicate that lesions within the transformation zone are usually more severe than those in the area of the original squamous epithelium. This even holds true for the mosaics and punctations arising within the transformation zone, which are most likely virally induced, and strongly suggests that these lesions arose via atypical basal hyperplasia.

Thus, there are two completely different types of mosaics and punctations: those within and those outside the transformation zone. They differ in their morphogenesis and in their "malignancy index." In the cases in our study, all of which contained CIN, this index was relatively high regardless of the localization of the lesions. It would have been considerably lower if all mosaics and punctations had been examined. If colposcopy is pursued routinely (as opposed to only in patients with abnormal cytology), a number of patients are seen in whom mosaic, punctation, and leukoplakia are merely acanthotic epithelium. Thus, the overall malignancy index of these lesions is only about 19% (6). But if colposcopy is used only to evaluate patients with abnormal cervical cytology, mosaics and punctations are seen mainly with CIN and the exceptions to the supposed rule—patients with abnormal colposcopy findings but benign histology—are puzzling.

These results should prompt a reevaluation of colposcopic diagnostics and of the morphogenesis of atypical epithelial changes at the cervix.

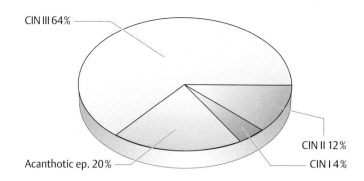

Fig. 10.**11** Histologic correlates of mosaics and punctations inside the transformation zone (25 lesions in 116 cases)

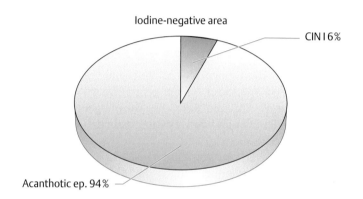

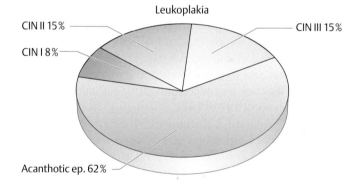

Fig. 10.**12** Histologic correlates of iodine-negative areas and leukoplakias in 87 cases

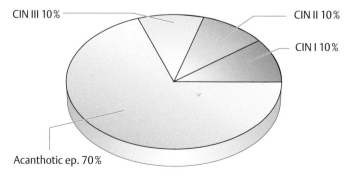

Fig. 10.**10** Histologic correlates of mosaics and punctations outside the transformation zone in 87 patients

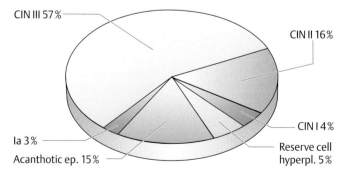

Fig. 10.**13** Topography of mosaic, punctation, leukoplakia, and iodine-negative areas in 118 cases (152 lesions)

References

1 Bajardi F. Colposcopic findings and their histologic correlates. Geburtshilfe Frauenheilkd 1984;44:84.

2 Burghardt E. Gibt es ein Flächenwachstum des intraepithelialen Carcinoms an der Cervix? Arch Gynäkol 1973;215:1.

3 Burghardt E. Premalignant lesions of the cervix. Clin Obstet Gynecol 1976;3:257.

4 Burghardt E. The importance of the last cervical gland in the natural history of cervical neoplasia. Obstet Gynecol Surv 1979;34:862.

5 Burghardt E, Östör AG. Site of origin and growth pattern of cervical cancer: a histomorphological study. Obstet Gynecol 1983;62:117.

6 Coppleson LW, Brown B. Estimation of the screening error rate from the observed detection rates in repeated cervical cytology. Am J Obstet Gynecol 1974;119:953–957.

7 Coppleson M, Reid BL. Preclinical carcinoma of the cervix uteri: its origin, nature and management. Oxford: Pergamon, 1967.

8 Girardi F. The topography of abnormal colposcopy findings. Cervix and lower female genital tract 1993;11:45–52.

9 Glatthaar E. Studium über die Morphogenese des Plattenepithelkarzinoms der Portio vaginalis uteri. Basel: Karger, 1950.

10 Hinselmann H. Ausgewählte Gesichtspunkte zur Beurteilung des Zusammenhanges der "Matrixbezirke" und des Karzinoms der sichtbaren Abschnitte des weiblichen Genitaltraktes. Z.Geburtsh 1933;104:228–252.

11 Homesley HD, Jobson VW, Reish RL. Use of colposcopically directed, four-quadrant cervical biopsy by the colposcopy trainee. J Reprod Med 1984;29:311.

12 Johnson LD, Driscoll SG, Hertig AT, Cole PT, Nickerson RJ. Vaginal adenosis in stillborns and neonates exposed to diethystilbestrol and steroidal estrogens and progestins. Obstet Gynecol 1979;53:671.

13 Kohan S, Noumoff J, Beckman EM, Morris M, Weiner E, Douglas GW. Colposcopic screening of women with atypical Papanicolaou smears. J Reprod Med 1985;30:279–285.

14 Navratil E. Colposcopy. In: Gray LA, ed. Dysplasia, carcinoma in situ and microinvasive carcinoma of the cervix . Springfield, IL: Thomas 1964:228.

15 Stafl A, Wilbanks G. An international terminology of colposcopy. Report of the nomenclature committee of the International Federation of Cervical Pathology and Coloposcopy. Obstet Gynecol 1991; 77:313–4.

16 Treite P. Die Frühdiagnose des Plattenepithel-Karzinoms am Collum uteri. Stuttgart: Enke, 1944.

11 Documenting Colposcopic Findings

Accurate documentation of colposcopic findings enables precise correlation of the colposcopic and histologic topography. Such comparisons, based on examination of properly processed conization specimens, are particularly useful for analyzing colposcopic appearances. Also, long-term observation of patients in whom each finding has been fully documented allows study of the dynamics of all the benign and atypical changes that take place on the cervix. Long-term follow-up studies are a challenge for future colposcopists. To date, there is no well-documented case, for example, of the development of intraepithelial neoplasia from an ectopy or original squamous epithelium while under observation. Such studies will contribute significantly to the understanding of the genesis of cervical carcinoma.

Colpophotography

Most colposcopes are fitted with photographic equipment (see Fig. 1.**3**). The camera is constructed so that the plane of the film coincides with that of vision. Fine focusing for the colposcopic examination serves the same purpose for photography. The flash used for illumination makes possible the shortest exposure time and the greatest depth of field. New developments, such as halogen lamps, ultrasensitive film, and automatic light meters produce high-quality pictures.

The quality of the colpophotograph depends to a large extent on the know-how and experience of the colposcopist. Although the pictures that appear in textbooks or in slide sets are good, they usually represent selections from much larger collections. Furthermore, they often show only a detail, and do not reflect the technical difficulties that may be encountered if larger lesions or the whole cervix are to be reproduced. It is not possible to portray faithfully each and every colposcopic lesion, so an accurate colposcopic diagnosis cannot be made merely from a colpophotograph. This problem, however, has been solved by other means (see below).

A special difficulty pertaining to colpophotography is the imperfect depth of field. If we think of the cervix as hemisphere, it becomes understandable how difficult it is to telescope into the one plane the images of lesions that cover the entire surface. The larger a lesion, the more difficult it is to photograph.

Another technical problem with colpophotography is the ubiquitous presence of highlights. They appear in the most unexpected places, especially if a flash is used. Using specula with nonreflective surfaces was unsuccessful in eliminating this.

Stereocolpophotography has not overcome these problems but is suitable for teaching purposes. A three-dimensional representation can be obtained by using a stereoviewer that depicts the surface relief of colposcopic lesions particularly well. Unfortunately, the picture can be seen by only one person at a time, and cannot be used in lectures.

Colpophotography normally employs color film. Black-and-white photography is useful to highlight certain details such as blood vessels. A green filter is particularly good for contrasting blood vessels. Fine-grained, orthochromatic film is recommended.

Other Photographic Equipment

The Kolpophot

In 1953, Ganse (4) developed the Kolpophot to photograph the cervix directly and not through the colposcope. A further technical advance was made by Baader (1, 3) from Freiburg, who started off with 35-mm photography but later replaced it with 60-mm (Rollei SL66). A combination of Zeiss-Planar S 120 and a ring flash with pilot light achieved excellent results. Magnification of ×1.5 was used, allowing reproduction of areas measuring up to 4 by 4 cm, which meant that even large cervices up to 4 cm in diameter could be reproduced (Fig. 11.**1**). With a light-sensitive film and a small aperture, a most satisfactory depth of field was achieved (Fig. 11.**2**).

The pictures produced by Baader cannot be bettered even by very high magnification. Using this technique, Baader addressed comparative colposcopy and colposcopic follow-up studies (3) better than anyone else. His incredible collection comprises, among others, adolescents who have been followed photographically over many years (3). A problem with this method is its clumsiness: as opposed to colpophotography, which can be performed at the same time as the colposcopic examination, Baader's method is a completely separate procedure.

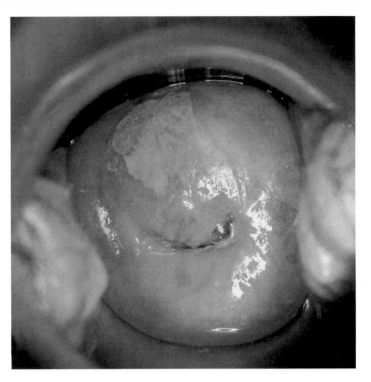

Fig. 11.**1**   Using special photography, the entire cervix can be reproduced (courtesy of O. Baader)

Cervicography

This technique was pioneered by Stafl (6, 7). According to Stafl, cervicography is not a substitute for colposcopy, only for colposcopic screening. This statement reinstates colposcopy to its original place. Colposcopy has always been regarded as part of the routine gynecologic examination, and as a screening method it should contribute to the early detection of cervical carcinoma. After the widespread adoption of cytology, colposcopy was relegated in many places to the visualization and localization of atypical changes suspected by cytology. Elsewhere, especially in Europe, cytology was always combined with colposcopy, as described in Chapter 12. This practice requires each gynecologist to be his or her own colposcopist.

Cervicography has a place in countries where gynecologists do not have sufficient colposcopic training. The camera devised by Stafl (National Testing Laboratories, St. Louis, Missouri) should enable anybody to take excellent photographs.

Cervicography had to overcome the technical problem of achieving satisfactory magnification from a working distance of at least 15 cm. A system was devised using a 100-mm lens attached to a 35-mm camera body with a 50-mm extension ring. To achieve constant magnification, the focusing ring of the lens is permanently fixed to 0.9 m. A ring strobe light is attached to the front lens of the objective. The cervicograph is focused by moving the entire system back and forth.

The cervicogram should be interpreted by experts. The cervicograph slide is projected on a screen 3 m or greater in width and observed from a distance of approximately 1 m. The apparent magnification is comparable to direct visual colposcopic magnification of ×11.

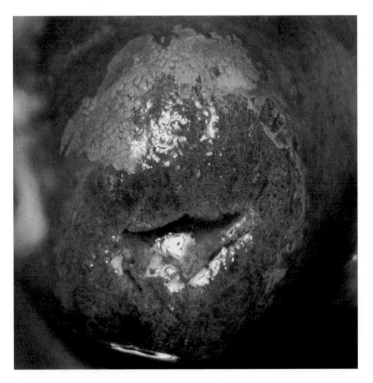

Fig. 11.**2**   The depth of field provided by special techniques allows photography of the cervix with the adjacent fornix (courtesy of O. Baader)

Cases of CIN were detected by this method, that were missed by cytology (8). However, the reported discrepancy between cervicography and cytology is unduly wide (see Table 12.**2**).

Graphic Representation of Colposcopic Findings

Because of the difficulties with photography described above the colposcopist needs a simple method to record findings. This can be achieved by a simple sketch to accompany the written description. A form with a schematic representation of the cervix is useful. The cervix is shown as a circle with a small horizontal oval in the center to signify the external os (Fig. 11.**3**). Either a preprinted form or a rubber stamp may be used. The lesions can then be drawn in detail.

The various colposcopic findings are represented by symbols agreed on by most authors (Fig. 11.**3**). The findings are further designated by abbreviations (Table 11.**1**). The various phases of transformation can be conveniently represented by several combinations of letters. The drawing itself can be annotated with the abbreviations, with arrows pointing to each area (Fig. 11.**3**). Such drawings are particularly impressive when the result of the Schiller test is added (Fig. 11.**3**); if a red pencil is used, even the various shades of brown can be indicated.

Table 11.**1** Abbreviations for colposcopic findings

Diagnosis	Abbreviation
Ectopy	E
Transformation zone	TZ
Ectopy with early transformation	EET
Transformation zone with ectopic rests	TZER
Gland openings	GO
Nabothian follicles	NF
Inconspicuous iodine-yellow area	IINA
Leukoplakia	L
Mosaic	M
Coarse mosaic	CM
Punctation	P
Coarse punctation	CP
White epithelium (atypical transformation zone)	WE
Cuffed gland openings	CGO
Atypical vessels	AV
True erosion	TE
Condyloma	C

References

1   Baader O. Colposcopic findings in contraception. J Reprod Med 1974;12:186.
2   Baader O. Probleme der Kolposkopie. Gynäkol Praxis 1982;6:91.
3   Baader O. Kolpophotographische Studien. Gynäkol Praxis 1982;6:101.
4   Ganse R. Kolpophotogramme zur Einführung in die Kolposkopie. 2 vols. Berlin: Akademie, 1953.
5   Ganse R. Über die Gefäßdarstellung kolposkopischer Befunde mit der Quecksilberdampflampe und dem Kolpophot. Zentralbl Gynäkol 1954:76:81.
6   Stafl A. Cervicography: a new approach to cervical cancer detection. Gynecol Oncol 1981;12:292.
7   Stafl A. Cervicography: a new method for cervical cancer detection. Am J Obstet Gynecol 1981;139:815.
8   Tawa K, Forsythe A, Cove JK, Saltz A, Peters WH, Watring WG. A comparison of the Papanicolau smear and the cervigram: sensitivity, specificity, and cost analysis. Obstet Gynecol 1988;71:229.

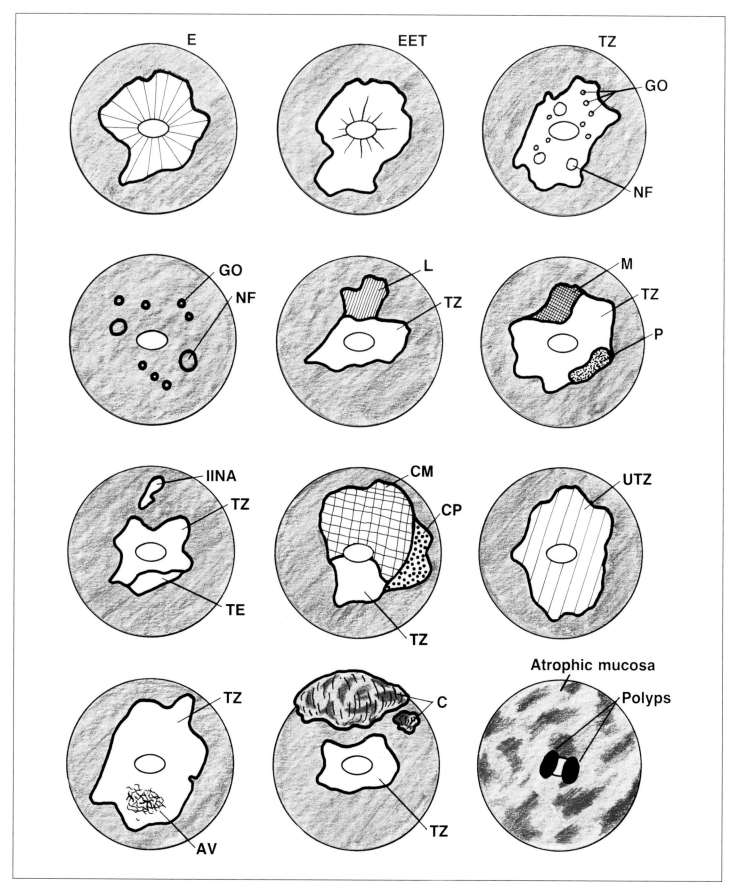

Fig. 11.**3 Graphic documentation of colposcopic findings.** It is easy to draw the contours of the various changes on a preprinted form and to indicate their nature using symbols and cross-hatching. Abbreviations can also be added (Table 11.**1**). Finally, the result of the Schiller test can be indicated with a red pencil

12

Uses of Colposcopy

Colposcopy can be applied (a) as an integral part of every gynecologic examination in concert with cytology; (b) to identify and localize lesions suspected on the basis of abnormal cytologic findings; and (c) to clarify the nature of clinically suspicious lesions.

Routine Colposcopy

This is by far the most appropriate application of colposcopy. Inspection of the cervix, vagina, and vulva is an essential part of the gynecologic examination. It stands to reason that such lesions are better seen when magnified and optimally illuminated. This is true for inflammatory lesions, polyps, and small fistulas as well as for preinvasive and early invasive neoplastic lesions. Properly taught and practiced, colposcopy should not be too time-consuming. Selective use of the colposcope does not make sense to the physician accustomed to using it routinely.

Colposcopy to Evaluate Abnormal Cervical Cytology

Using colposcopy to evaluate only patients with abnormal cytologic findings has several drawbacks. First, the colposcopist will see only selected, nonrepresentative cases. There will be gaps that make it more difficult to understand normal and abnormal developments that take place at the cervix. In contrast, routine colposcopy facilitates an appreciation of the dynamic processes that occur at the cervix in the different phases of life. It is very illuminating to follow a given patient over the years. Also, the colposcopist will come to appreciate the morphogenesis of CIN. Ignorance of facets of cervical dynamics will lead to wrong conclusions and misconceptions.

Second, selective colposcopy precludes the opportunity to pick up abnormalities missed by cytologic screening. The accuracy of cytologic diagnoses can be determined only by routine histology, which is neither indicated nor appropriate, or by a second screening method. Colposcopy is easy to combine with routine cytology. The diagnostic accuracy of cytology and colposcopy can then be checked by biopsying all colposcopically suspect findings (Table 12.**1**). In the absence of such quality control, the accuracy of cytology will be overestimated. Even good cytologic laboratories can have false negative rates of up to 20%, partly due to inadequate smears (2, 6, 9, 13, 15–19). Only a second screening modality can compensate for these errors.

Third, if colposcopy is not used routinely it will be regarded as cumbersome and time-consuming. With practice, the colposcopist can reach a quick and accurate diagnosis of visible lesions. Experienced colposcopists are consistently surprised by the ado concerning colposcopy at institutions where the procedure is performed only for selected patients. This practice gives the procedure a reputation of being costly, cumbersome, and time-consuming.

Colposcopy to Evaluate Clinically Suspicious Lesions

This implies using colposcopy to clarify the nature of cervical changes seen with the naked eye. This practice is superior to colposcopy restricted to evaluating abnormal smears because it can pick up some lesions missed by cytology. But it is not as effective as routine colposcopy because it will miss lesions not picked up by gross inspection of the cervix and because there is no opportunity to inspect the lower reaches of the cervical canal. Considering that only 15–20% of lesions are purely endocervical (3–5, 7, 11, 12, 14), not too much time is wasted by examining these cases. If colposcopy is limited to evaluating grossly suspicious lesions, then its role is merely to avoid unnecessary biopsies.

Table 12.**1** Colposcopic and cytologic findings in 838 cases of histologically proven carcinoma in situ and microinvasive carcinoma (10)

Method of detection	Cases
Colposcopy	663 (79%)
Cytology	729 (87%)
Colposcopy and cytology	828 (99%)

Cytology and Colposcopy

Both cytology and colposcopy are primarily screening methods to detect early cervical cancer. Cytology provides a snapshot of the changes taking place at the cervix at any one time. Colposcopy also allows study of the natural history of physiologic processes at the cervix and assessment of the development of any given abnormality. Both methods are associated with error rates. Mistakes in cytology can result from poor smears or from misinterpreting them. Colposcopic failures are due to misinterpreting changes and to the fact that lesions in the canal can be out of reach of the colposcope. As the diagnostic principles of the two methods are quite different, it is unlikely that a lesion will be missed if both methods are used in concert (1, 4, 10, 11, 19).

Cytology is undoubtedly more accurate than colposcopy, and should be the method of choice if only one method is available. As its success does not depend on the location of a lesion, well-taken smears should reveal abnormalities in the canal at the same rate as those on the ectocervix. Cytology has a failure rate, the reasons for which are not always clear. The false-negative rate is stated to be between 5% and 30% (see above). The wide range cannot be attributed merely to differing degrees of competence among the various observers. It also results from the type of quality control. Colposcopy is particularly suitable as a second screening method to compensate for cytologic failures (1, 4, 10, 11, 20).

The failure rate of colposcopy must be higher than that of good cytology screening, simply because 10–15% of atypical lesions are situated in the canal, out of range of the colposcope (see above). To this must be added a further 5% due to misinterpretation of ectocervical changes. It is therefore reasonable to regard colposcopy as 80% accurate in the detection of early cervical carcinoma (1, 4, 8, 10, 11, 16).

Table 12.**2** shows how the two methods complement each other in the diagnosis of carcinoma in situ and microinvasive carcinoma. Both modalities were positive in only 220 of 306 cases. Conversely, in only 4 cases (1.3%) were both colposcopy and cytology negative. Although cytology detected 51 more cases than colposcopy, 31 cases would have been missed had colposcopy not been performed (10).

These are the best results that can be achieved. The cytologic examinations were performed only by cytopathologists. With widespread cytologic screening by personnel with less training the failure rate must be higher. If colposcopy is reserved only for the evaluation of abnormal smears, the failure rate is built in, the detection rate cannot be improved, and the usefulness of colposcopy is diminished.

Table 12.**2** Cytologic and colposcopic findings in 306 cases of histologically proven carcinoma in situ and microinvasive carcinoma (10)

Finding	Cases
Cytology positive – Colposcopy positive	220 (72%)
Cytology negative – Colposcopy positive	26 (8.5%)
Cytology unsatisfactory – Colposcopy positive	5 (2%)
Cytology positive – Colposcopy negative	51 (17%)
Cytology negative – Colposcopy negative	4 (1%)
Detected by both methods	302 (99%)

Colposcopically Directed Cytology

In contrast to cytology, colposcopy can localize suspicious lesions. Even if the ectocervix is colposcopically normal but the cytology is positive, an endocervical lesion may be safely predicted, provided the vagina and fornices are normal. In this way, cytology can select patients for biopsy.

Conversely, it is possible to direct the cytology smear under colposcopic control. Thus, a colposcopic lesion can be scraped directly with an Ayre's spatula, or the endocervical canal can be carefully sampled when there are no lesions on the ectocervix. The reliability of cytology under these circumstances must be much greater than random sampling with the naked eye. There is no doubt that the quality of cytology can be improved by the simultaneous use of colposcopy.

Routine Combination of Colposcopy and Cytology

To achieve the best possible diagnosis of early cervical cancer, colposcopy can be routinely combined with cytology in two different ways:

1. A smear is taken at the time of colposcopy, and biopsy of any suspicious lesion is done at the same time without waiting for the result of cytology. In this way a false-negative cytologic result is compensated by colposcopy and biopsy. This practice can have several outcomes:

– Colposcopy and biopsy positive, cytology positive
– Colposcopy and biopsy positive, cytology negative
– Colposcopy positive, biopsy negative, cytology positive

In this case, another area must undergo biopsy. If the latter is again negative, which is unusual, and the cytology is unequivocal, conization is indicated.

– Colposcopy positive, biopsy negative, cytology negative

In such cases, colposcopic and cytologic follow-up, and even repeat biopsy, are recommended.

2. In spite of colposcopically suspicious lesions, biopsy is deferred until the result of cytology is known. If cytology is normal, repeat smears should be taken, and the cytologist warned of the colposcopist's findings. In the rare instance of persistently normal cytologic findings in association with highly suspicious colposcopy, biopsy is indicated.

One final combination may result from the simultaneous application of colposcopy and cytology:

– Colposcopy negative, cytology positive

In this case colposcopy should be repeated, and even a suspicious lesion at the ectocervix should be biopsied. In addition, the endocervical canal should be thoroughly curetted. If histology is normal and cytology remains abnormal, the biopsy should be repeated, or conization carried out. It should be remembered that the vagina can also be the source of abnormal cytologic findings.

References

1 Bajardi F, Burghardt E, Kern H, Kroemer H. Nouveaux résultats de la cytologie et de la colposcopie systématiques dans le diagnostique précoce du cancer du col de l'utérus. Gynécol Prat 1959;5:315.

2 Bayrle W. Kritische Betrachtungen zur Rate der "falsch negativen" Befunde in der gynäkologischen Zytologie. Geburtshilfe Frauenheilkd 1977;37:864.

3 Burghardt E. Early histological diagnosis of cervical cancer. Philadelphia: Saunders, 1973.

4 Burghardt E, Bajardi F. Ergebnisse der Früherfassung des Collumcarcinoms mittels Cytologie und Kolposkopie an der Univ.-Frauenklinik Graz 1954. Arch Gynäkol 1956;187:621.

5 Burghardt E, Holzer E. Die Lokalisation des pathologischen Cervixepithels, 1: Carcinoma in situ, Dysplasien und abnormes Plattenepithel. Arch Gynäkol 1970;209:305.

6 Coppleson LW, Brown B. Estimation of the screening error rate from the observed detection rates in repeated cervical cytology. Am J Obstet Gynecol 1974;119:953.

7 Kern G. Carcinoma in situ. Berlin: Springer, 1964.

8 Kolstadt P. Colposcopic diagnosis of cervical neoplasia. In: Jordan AJ, Singer A. The cervix. Philadelphia: Saunders, 1976:36–411.

9 Naujoks H, Leppien G, Rogosaroff-Fricke R. Negativer zytologischer Abstrich bei Carcinoma in situ der Cervix uteri. Geburtshilfe Frauenheilkd 1976;36:570.

10 Navratil E. Colposcopy. In: Gray LA, ed. Dysplasia, carcinoma in situ and microinvasive carcinoma of the cervix uteri. Springfield, IL: Thomas, 1964:10–228.

11 Navratil E, Burghardt E, Bajardi F, Nash W. Simultaneous colposcopy and cytology used in screening for carcinoma of the cervix. Am J Obstet Gynecol 1958;75:1292.

12 Ober KG, Bontke E. Sitz und Ausdehnung der Carcinomata in situ und der beginnenden Krebse der Cervix. Arch Gynäkol 1959;192:55.

13 Pederson E, Hoeg H, Kolstadt P. Mass screening for cancer of the uterine cervix in Ostfold County, Norway: an experiment. Second report of the Norwegian Cancer Society. Acta Obstet Gynecol Scand 1971; suppl 11.

14 Reagan JW, Pattern F Jr. Dysplasia: a basic reaction to injury in the uterine cervix. Ann NY Acad Sci 1962;97:662.

15 Rylander E. Negative smears in women developing invasive cervical cancer. Acta Obstet Gynecol Scand 1977;56:115.

16 Seidl S. Praktische Karzinom-Frühdiagnostik in der Gynäkologie. Stuttgart: Thieme, 1974.

17 Seybolt JF, Johnson WD. Cervical cytodiagnostic problems: a survey. Am J Obstet Gynecol 1971;109:1089.

18 Shingleton WP, Rutledge R. To cone or not to cone the cervix. Obstet Gynecol 1968;31:430.

19 Stafl A, Friedrich EG, Mattingly RF. Detection of cervical neoplasia: reducing the risk of error. Clin Obstet Gynecol 1973;16:238.

20 Walker EM, Dodgson J, Duncan ID. Does mild atypia on a cervical smear warrant further investigation? Lancet 1986;11:672.

13

Colposcopy of the Vulva

Anatomy

The vulva is covered by two types of squamous epithelium. Peripherally keratinizing epidermis covers the mons pubis, the labia majora, and the sulci interlabiales to the labia minora. The inner aspects of the labia minora have no hair but do have talc, sweat and apocrine glands. Centrally the epidermis borders on the nonkeratinizing glycogen-containing squamous epithelium of the vaginal vestibulum (Fig. 13.1). The squamous epithelium of the vulva, particularly the glycogen-containing mucous membranes, is very sensitive to hormonal influences. The border between the keratinized and nonkeratinized epithelia is called Hart's line. It is sometimes visible to the naked eye but is always visible microscopically (1). Hart's line is best seen at the posterior fourchette, and it marks the peripheral border of the vaginal vestibulum. The vaginal vestibulum comprises the outer aspect of the hymen, the frenulum clitoridis, the inner aspect of the labia minora, the vaginal introitus, and the external urethral orifice.

The vulva can be affected by dermatologic conditions and by specific conditions. The vulva is an epithelial high-risk area with a predisposition to multifocal and recurrent malignant transformation.

The epidermis is a stratified squamous epithelium composed of distinct layers. In a vertical section the epidermis has an undulating appearance caused by the malpighian rete. The deepest layer, resting on the basement membrane, is the basal cell layer (germinative layer, stratum germinativum) from which the epithelium regenerates. The basal cells are undifferentiated and pluripotent. The basal layer also contains melanocytes, which are highly differentiated. The spinal cell layer (stratum spinosum) is the layer most variable in thickness. The next layer, the granular layer (stratum granulosum), is followed by the horny layer (stratum corneum), which also varies in thickness.

The glycogen-containing mucous membrane of the introitus and the vagina has the same appearances as the cervical epithelium and is very sensitive to hormonal influences. With the lack of estrogen in childhood and after menopause, this layer consists of few layers and is thus thin and easily injured. The effects of the sexual hormones gives the characteristic multilayered appearance. Apart from the basal cell layer, which does not contain melanocytes, the next cell layers are pretty uniform. All contain glycogen in the cytoplasm, which makes the epithelium look honeycombed in hematoxylin-eosin sections. Apart from the basal cell layer one can distinguish only an intermediate and a superficial cell layer.

Diagnostic Methods for Vulvar Lesions

(Table 13.1)

History. A detailed history is often difficult to obtain from patients with conditions of the vulva. In younger patients the history is often closely related to the often acute condition, whereas older patients generally have chronic lesions. Some older patients are forgetful and have become accustomed to their condition. The discrepancy between subjective complaints and the objective findings is often marked.

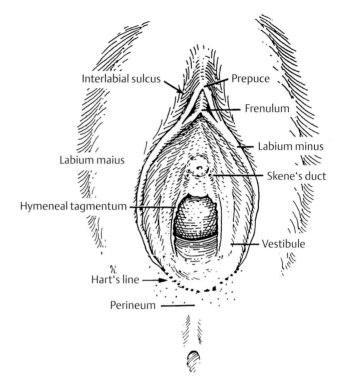

Fig. 13.**1 Topography of the vulva** and the perineum with Hart's line

Table 13.**1** Diagnostic methods for lesions of the vulva

Clinical methods
    History
    Inspection
    Palpation
    Photography (including digital image analysis)
    Toluidine blue test (Collins test)
    Acetic acid test
    Colposcopy
    Colpophotography (with digital image analysis)

Laboratory methods
    Biopsy (punch biopsy, excisional biopsy)
    Exfoliative cytology
    DNA hybridization techniques for human papillomavirus

Characteristic symptoms of vulvar lesions are pruritus, burning sensations, paresthesias, and dyspareunia. The relevant surgical, medical (diabetes), and psychiatric history should be elicited. Medications, estrogen replacement, allergies, incontinence, and prior vaginitis and sexually transmitted diseases are of interest.

Inspection. A number of conditions can be diagnosed with confidence by inspection only. These include malformations, traumatic lesions, cysts, certain tumors and ulcers, papillomas, condylomas, atrophy, and lichen sclerosus et atrophicus (LSA). However, many vulvar conditions vary in appearance, and sometimes multiple conditions overlap. In these cases diagnoses should be made with caution or with the support of other tests.

Grossly, lesions of the vulva can be classified according to color as red (erythroplakia), white (leukoplakia), or pigmented (melanotic) lesions. Colposcopy is often helpful to distinguish between these and to obtain a representative biopsy sample.

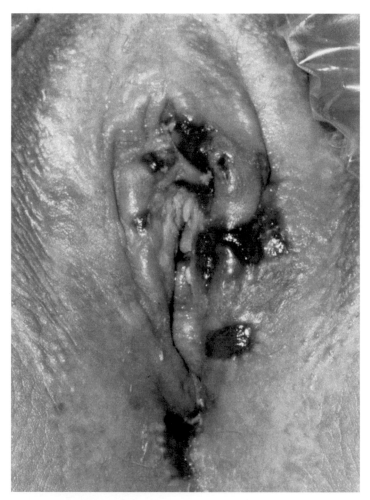

Fig. 13.**2** **Multicentric, sharply demarcated foci of VIN 3.** Note the marked red color before application of toluidine blue

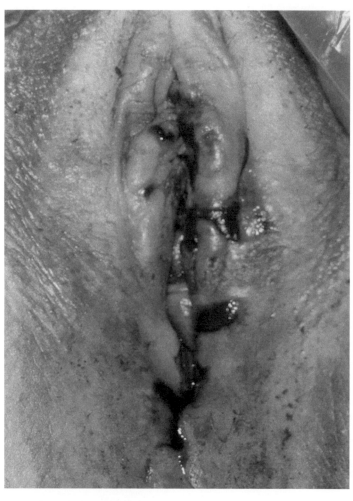

Fig. 13.**3** **Positive toluidine blue stain in the areas with VIN 3.** The lichen sclerosus et atrophicus (LSA) does not stain

Vulvar lesions that do not resolve within weeks have to be followed closely to detect progression. Pure description is inadequate in these cases because it is subjective and poorly reproducible even by the same examiner. These cases should be documented with photography.

Palpation. Most vulvar conditions, whether raised from the surrounding tissue or not, are normal to palpation. However, even small invasive carcinomas show a tougher consistency around their base than the surrounding tissue. Small invasive foci can be detected in large areas of high-grade VIN (vulvar intraepithelial neoplasia) by palpation alone. When these lesions grow, they are no longer at the level of the surrounding tissue and become less mobile against the dermis.

Toluidine blue test (Collins test). One percent toluidine blue solution is applied to the vulva for 2–3 minutes and then washed off with 1% acetic acid. This method is a native stain for cell nuclei, which can be increased in neoplastic lesions or exposed in ulcers. Thus, a positive result of this test is unspecific (Figs. 13.**2**, 13.**3**). A negative result—i.e., the absence of staining or after destaining by acetic acid—makes a malignant lesion unlikely. The toluidine blue test can also be used during surgery to plan the margins of the excision. However, the test has become almost obsolete with the increased use of colposcopy with the application of acetic acid (see p. 20). This method shows much more detail for colposcopy, particularly papillary lesions and the typical findings of punctations and mosaics (Fig. 13.**4**).

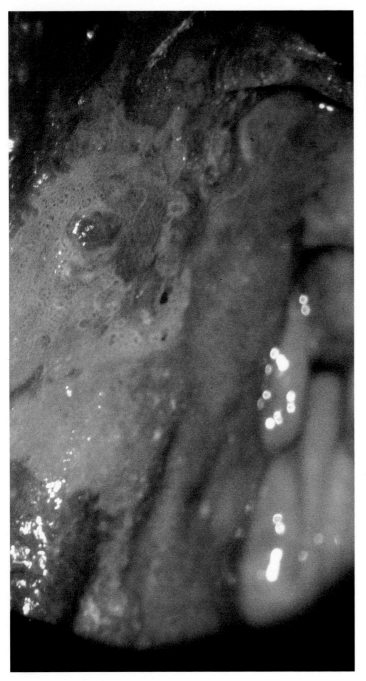

Fig. 13.**4** **VIN 3 after application of acetic acid.** There is marked punctation and a slight mosaic

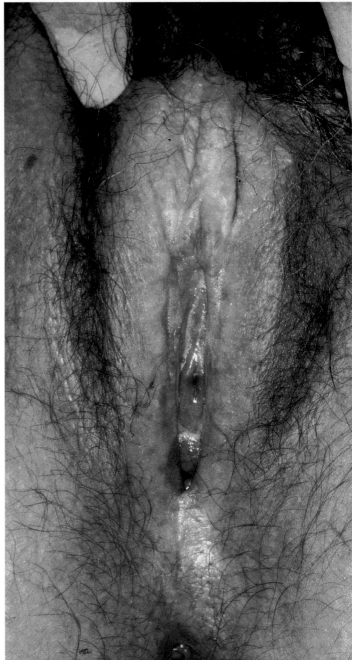

Fig. 13.**5** **Pale epidermis with LSA**

Colposcopy of the Vulva

The magnification of a colposcope permits more precise evaluation and earlier detection of epithelial lesions of the vulva than inspection with the naked eye. The color of a vulvar lesion depends on a number of factors.

Redness is caused by hypervascularization due to acute inflammation or a number of malignant lesions or their precursors. Redness can be circumscribed or diffuse.

Whiteness can be caused by dystrophic conditions such as lichen sclerosus et atrophicus which sclerose the stroma and decrease the blood supply (Fig. 13.**5**). *Leukoplakia* is a general

term for whitish lesion and is seen particularly with malignant conditions. In these lesions a thick cornified layer reflects light before it can reach the deeper layers or the stroma (Figs. 13.**6**, 13.**7**).

The melanocytes in the basal cell layer produce and contain melanin that produces dark brown to black color. Apart from the marked lesions of malignant melanoma and its precursors, about 30% of all high-grade VINs are associated with irregular hyperpigmentation (Fig. 13.**8**).

Erythroplakia is a general descriptive term for reddish lesions and is caused by a dense collection of atypical blood vessels. Erythroplakia is characteristic for premalignant or malig-

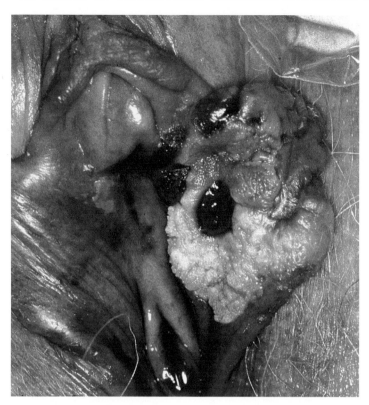

Fig. 13.**6 Cockade-like appearance of a wide high-grade** VIN with squamous leukoplakia and an erythroplakic center

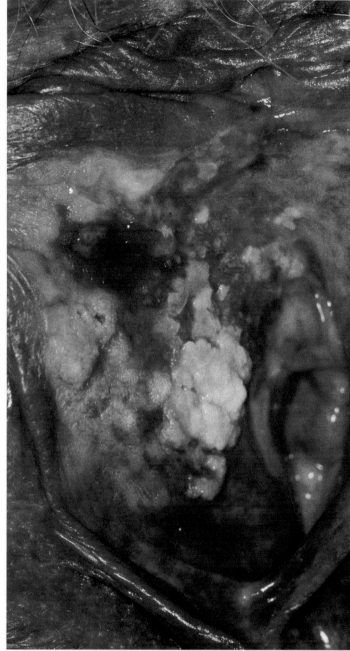

Fig. 13.**7 Cockade-like appearance of a wide high-grade VIN** with squamous leukoplakia and an erythroplakic center

nant lesions (Fig. 13.**11**). Leukoplakia is also a general descriptive term for whitish lesions and is caused by a variable thickening of the superficial keratinized epithelial layers (Figs. 13.**9**, 13.**10**). Both leukoplakia and erythroplakia are very similar to those at the cervix and appear under the colposcope as mosaics and punctations (see pp. 54, 59) (Figs. 13.**9**–13.**11**). They are more common in the nonkeratinizing, glycogen-containing squamous epithelium of the introitus than in the remaining vulva, where leukoplakic lesions are more common (Fig. 13.**12**).

An important feature at colposcopy of the vulva is how a lesion is contrasted from its surroundings. Abnormalities of the epithelium are usually sharply demarcated from their surrounding normal epithelium, as are different types of abnormal epithelia amongst themselves. In contrast, inflammation af-

fects the stroma more than the epithelium and its borders are much less defined. The feature of sharp demarcation applies especially to carcinomas of all sizes. An early cancer usually appears as erythroplakia either raised or lower than the surrounding tissue (Figs. 13.**9**, 13.**13**). On the other hand, most suspicious lesions show a wide glacis that consists of either abnormal epithelium such as LSA or a true premalignant condition such as VIN (Fig. 13.**14**). But here erythroplakic invasive areas can occur in the middle of noninvasive leukoplakic areas with VIN that can be considered border areas (Figs. 13.**6**, 13.**15**). Carcinomas without premalignant border zones lead to recurrent debates on the de novo theory of carcinogenesis. Primary leukoplakic carcinomas, which almost always are well-differentiated verrucous neoplasias, are much rarer (see Fig. 13.**23**).

Fig. 13.**8a**

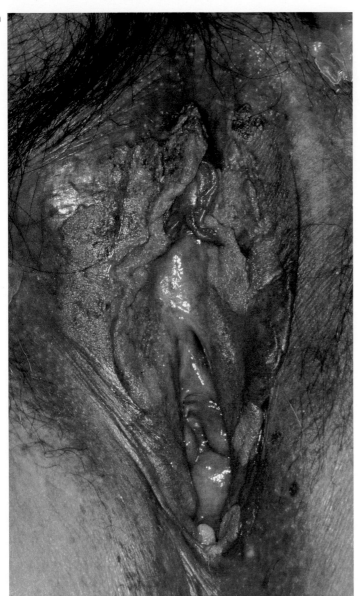

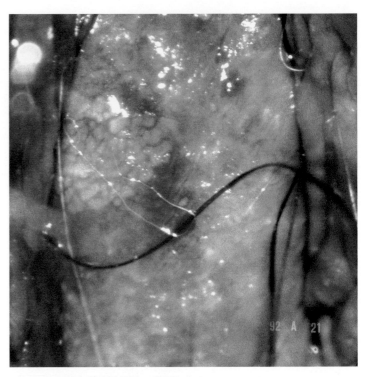

Fig. 13.**9** **Flat, raised carcinoma** with punctation and a sharp demarcation toward the mucosa of the vestibulum

Fig. 13.**8b**

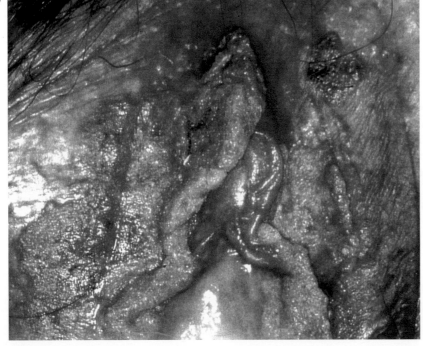

Fig. 13.**8a** **Bowenoid papillomatosis** with partial hyperpigmentation

Fig. 13.**8b** Colposcopic magnification

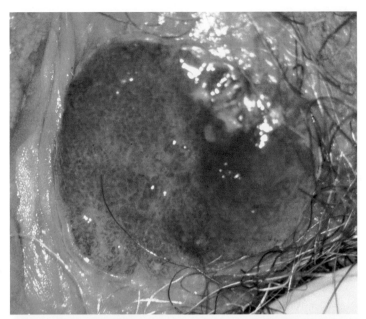

Fig. 13.**10**   **Marked mosaic** due to wide leukoplakic epithelial ridges

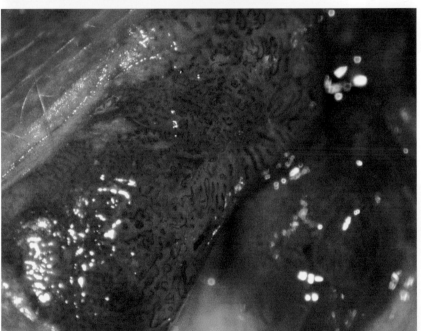

Fig. 13.**11**   **Marked vascular pattern of a mosaic.** Histology showed VIN 3 with microinvasion

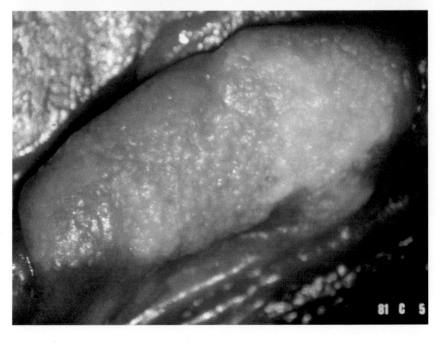

Fig. 13.**12**   **Sharply demarcated hyperkeratotic white lesion** corresponding to VIN 3

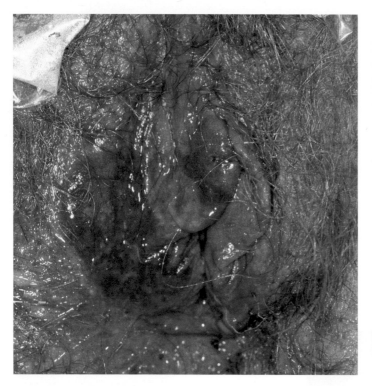

Fig. 13.**13**   **Sharply demarcated, slightly raised erythroplakic lesion** corresponding to bowenoid-warty VIN 3

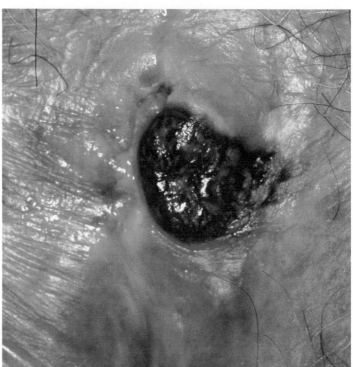

Fig. 13.**14**   **Flat microinvasive carcinoma** within LSA on the left side of the frenulum of the clitoris

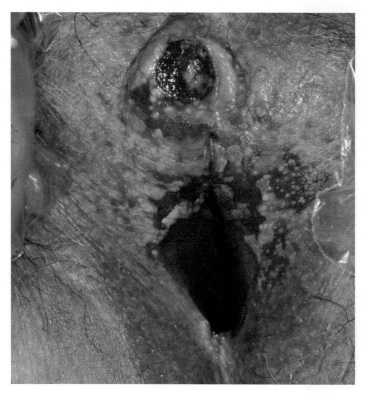

Fig. 13.**15**   **VIN 3 with erythroplakia and leukoplakia.** There is a sharply demarcated microinvasive carcinoma on the clitoris

Biopsy

All chronic lesions and acute conditions that do not resolve promptly should be biopsied. The indications for biopsy should be generous and should certainly not be limited to patients with abnormal cytology. All suspicious lesions, whether white, gray, red, pigmented, or raised, should be biopsied (2). Biopsies can be performed quickly and simply with local anesthesia on an outpatient basis with just a few instruments (Fig. 13.**16**).

Exfoliative Cytology

Cytologic smears provide adequate results in only about half of suspicious lesions. Biopsy is far superior to cytology (3).

Diagnosis of HPV Infection

HPV infection can be diagnosed with a number of hybridization techniques (dot blot, sandwich, filter in situ, hybrid capture, polymerase chain reaction [PCR]). This permits differentiation between low-risk (HPV type 6 and 11) and high-risk (type 16 and 18) infections.

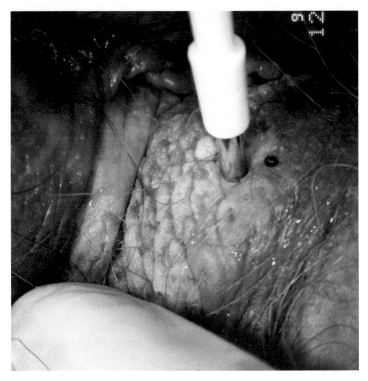

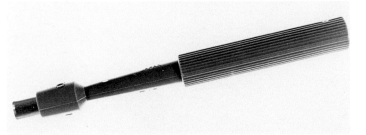

Fig. 13.**16 b**   The biopsy punch

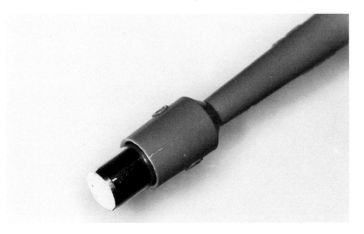

Fig. 13.**16 a–c**   **Punch biopsy**   Fig. 13.**16 a**   The biopsy punch at the vulva

Fig. 13.**16 c**   Magnification of the biopsy punch

Histologic Correlates of Colposcopic Findings

The normal epithelium of the vulva typically shows four histologic types: (1) glycogen-containing squamous epithelium proximal to Hart's line (within the introitus); (2) typical epidermis with or without acanthosis or hyperkeratosis; (3) lichenified squamous epidermis-type epithelium with epithelial atrophy and hyalinization of the upper dermis; and (4) atrophic squamous epithelium.

Apart from hyperkeratosis and leukoplakia in nonpathological epidermis, there are also erythroplakic areas in atrophic glycogen-containing squamous epithelium (Fig. 13.**17**). Hyperkeratotic leukoplakic areas in areas with lichen sclerosus et atrophicus suggest premalignant or malignant lesions (Fig. 13.**18**). All types of VIN can cause marked hyperkeratosis visible as leukoplakia.

Punctations and mosaics in nonmalignant lesions correspond to thin epithelial ridges and wide stromal papillae. In malignant lesions the stromal papillae are much narrower and the epithelial ridges plumper and more irregular. In vertical sections the differences between normal and atypical squamous epithelium are even more apparent. Papillae and papillary ridges of considerable height can be seen in hyperplastic epidermis as well as in all types of VIN.

High and thin stromal papillae in papillary, mild VIN are especially well seen. Papillomatous high-grade VINs often show marked but irregular stromal papillae.

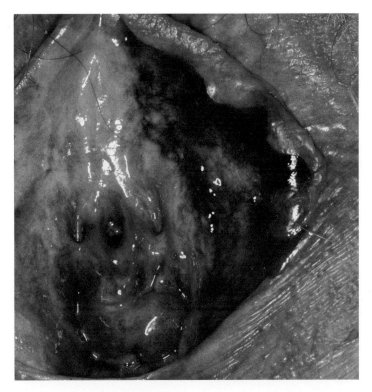

Fig. 13.**17**   **Atrophic vulvar skin with an erythroplakic lesion** that is indistinctly demarcated toward the vestibulum but sharply demarcated versus the left labium minus

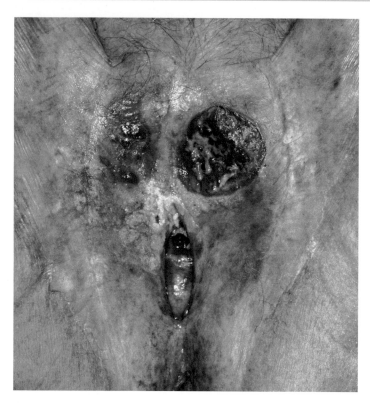

Fig. 13.**18** **LSA containing a deeply invasive carcinoma** on the left above the clitoris

Sharp and distinct borders between normal and abnormal epithelia are characteristic. The larger the difference in the differentiation of areas of adjoining VIN, the clearer the border between them.

Wide areas of papillomatosis can be caused by different degrees of VIN (Fig. 13.**19**). Large condylomata accuminata (Figs. 13.**20**, 13.**21**) and Buschke-Löwenstein type giant condylomas can harbor well-differentiated verrucous carcinomas (Figs. 13.**22**, 13.**23**). Condylomatous lesions can also be due to VIN III or squamous cell carcinomas.

Precursors of malignant melanomas regularly show dark gray to black pigmentation. In melanoma in situ the overlying epidermis can be hyperplastic and acanthotic (Fig. 13.**24**). The atypical pigmented melanocytes are in the basal cell layer or in the irregular clumps of cells in the upper dermis. *Invasive malignant melanomas* are usually dark brown to black (Fig. 13.**25**). Under the colposcope broad pigment network with dark brown and black globules and irregular extensions can be seen.

Paget's disease of the vulva characteristically forms sharp-bordered red or sometimes slightly whitish lesions only in the epidermal region (Fig. 13.**26**). In contrast to the uncharacteristically gross findings, the histologic appearance is typical. Clear cells are seen particularly in the basal cell layer, but also in more superficial layers of the epidermis. Heterotopic clear cells stem from adenocarcinomas in the deep layers of the dermis in apocrine and eccrine glands. This intraepithelial clear cell carcinoma induces epithelial hyperplasia with hyperkeratosis. Orthotopic Paget's disease is thought to be based on the embryonic multipotentiality of the basal cells (3).

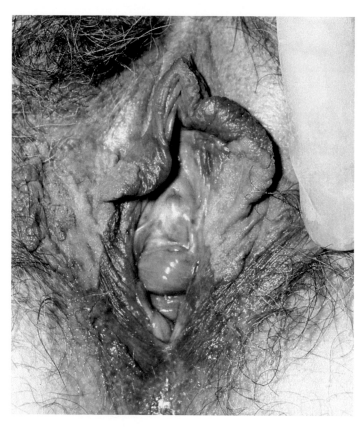

Fig. 13.**19 a** **Flat papillomatosis** in the right interlabial sulcus

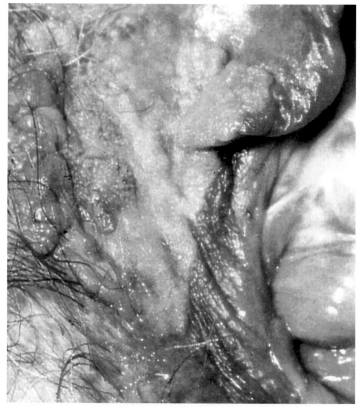

Fig. 13.**19 b** Colposcopic magnification

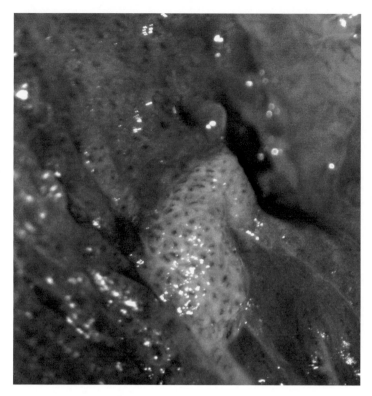

Fig. 13.**20**   Condyloma acuminatum with marked punctation

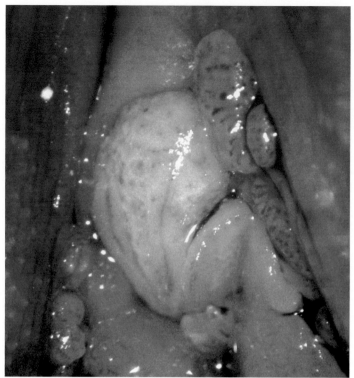

Fig. 13.**21**   **Marked papillomatosis** of the vulva with marked vascular patterns

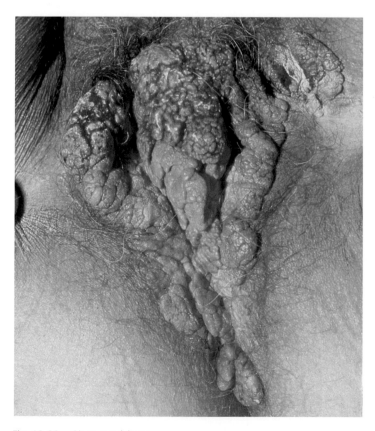

Fig. 13.**22**   Giant condyloma (Buschke-Löwenstein type) with malignant transformation

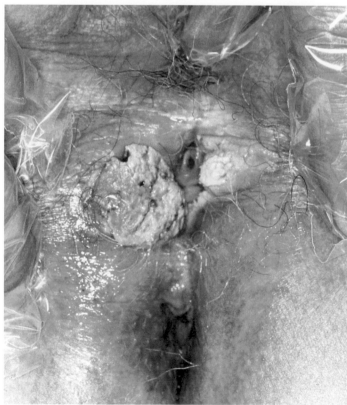

Fig. 13.**23**   **Verrucous vulvar carcinoma**

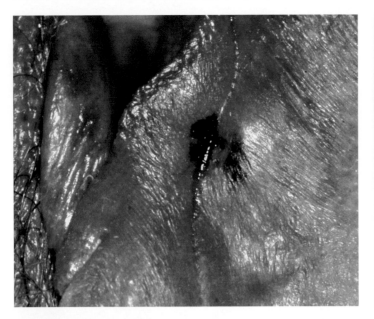

Fig. 13.**24** **Melanoma in situ**
in the left interlabial sulcus

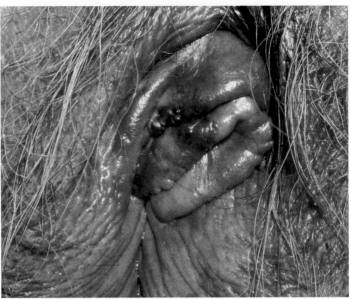

Fig. 13.**25** **Partially amelanotic
malignant melanoma** of the vulva

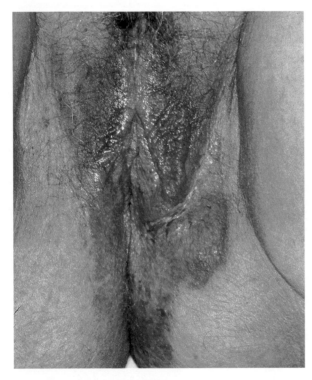

Fig. 13.**26** **Paget's disease** of the
vulva with sharply demarcated erythroplakia and leukoplakia on the
posterior region of the labia majora
and the perianal region

Table 13.**2** Classification of vulvar diseases according to International
Society for the Study of Vulvar Diseases (ISSVD) and the International
Society of Gynaecological Pathologists (ISGP)

I Nonneoplastic epithelial disorders of vulvar skin and mucosa
    – Lichen sclerosus (LS)
    – Squamous cell hyperplasia (formerly hyperplastic dystrophy)
    – Other dermatoses
    – Mixed epithelial disorders
    In such cases it is recommended the both conditions should be re-
    ported. For example, LS with associated squamous cell hyperplasia
    (formerly classified as mixed dystrophy) should be reported as LS
    and squamous cell hyperplasia. Squamous cell hyperplasia with as-
    sociated vulvar intraepithelial neoplasia (VIN) (formerly hyperplastic
    dystrophy with atypia) should be diagnosed as VIN.
    Squamous cell hyperplasia is used for those instances in which the
    hyperplasia is not attributable to another cause. Other dermatoses
    involving the vulva (e.g., psoriasis, lichen planus, lichen simplex
    chronicus, candida infection, condyloma acuminata) may include
    squamous cell hyperplasia but should be diagnosed specifically and
    excluded from this category.

II Neoplastic epithelial disorders of vulvar skin and mucosa (VIN)
    – Squamous intraepithelial neoplasia
      – VIN 1 (mild dysplasia)
      – VIN 2 (moderate dysplasia)
      – VIN 3 (severe dysplasia or carcinoma in situ)

III Nonsquamous intraepithelial neoplasia
    – Paget's disease
    – Melanoma in situ

Histologic Terminology and Classification

The International Society for the Study of Vulvar Diseases
(ISSVD) and the International Society of Gynaecological
Pathologists (ISGYP) have formulated a classification of vul-
var diseases with three major categories (4) (Table 13.**2**).

Colposcopy of the vulva is particularly useful for the following conditions:

1. Lichen sclerosus with its hypertrophic or atrophic forms,
   particularly with regard to concomitant VIN (see p. 160).
2. Erythroleukoplakic lesions of the keratinized and nonkeratinized glycogen-containing squamous epithelium. This includes most cases of VIN (see p. 158).

3. Precursors of and early malignant melanomas (p. 162).
4. Paget's disease of the vulva, which is also erythroleuko-plakic (p. 162).

The first three conditions occur both in the epidermis and in the glycogen-containing squamous epithelium; Paget's disease occurs only in the epidermis.

Gross Appearance of VIN

VIN is the most common neoplastic and preinvasive lesion of the vulvar epithelium. VIN can present as erythroplakia, leukoplakia, pigmented lesions, papulous lesions, and erosions and ulcers (5). This means that VIN can look like any of a number of benign dermatoses. VIN cannot be diagnosed reliably with colposcopy, and all suspicious lesions should be biopsied.

Histomorphology of VIN

All grades of VIN are precursors of squamous cell carcinomas of the vulva. The rate of progression of VIN to invasive carcinoma is 2–87%, ranging from 2–4% for low-grade to 87% for high-grade lesions (6). Vulvar carcinoma never develops directly from normal squamous cell epithelium; all carcinomas develop from VIN. Discrete lesions usually correspond to VIN 1 (mild dysplasia); more marked lesions usually correspond to VIN 2 (moderate dysplasia) or VIN 3 (severe dysplasia).

Kaufman (7) distinguished three major types of VIN:

1. *Undifferentiated or basaloid VIN.* Per definition this type of VIN consists exclusively of relatively uniform, small, and atypical cells that resemble the normal cells of the basal cell layer. They occupy almost the entire thickness of the epithelium. The most superficial layers can show signs of parakeratosis. Mitotic figures can be found in the entire epithelium except for the superficial layer.
2. *Bowenoid-warty VIN.* This type of VIN no longer shows the regularity of the basaloid type. The cell density is still high, but the cellular uniformity has given way to a more marked anisomorphy and anisokaryosis. Giant nuclei are present. The mitotic rate is high. Marked papillae are common, as the term "warty" implies. Hyperkeratosis and parakeratosis is common.
3. *Well-differentiated carcinoma in situ (simplex).* This used to be called high-grade VIN. It is characterized by a much lower nuclear density, mitoses are seen infrequently in the basal layer. There are also no marked nuclear atypias. There is only mild anisokaryosis, similar to CIN 1 and 2. The epithelium is usually thick and can show marked hyperkeratosis (more rarely parakeratosis).

These premalignant and malignant lesions, particularly all VINs regardless of HPV status, occur in more or less well demarcated fields. The basaloid and bowenoid types of VIN are usually seen in younger women and are associated with HPV type 16 infection. Well-differentiated carcinoma in situ is more common in older patients and is not associated with HPV infection (8).

Table 13.**3**   Treatment options for vulvar intraepithelial neoplasia (VIN)

1	Conservative management
2	Wide local excision using a knife or laser
3	Laser ablation
4	Medical therapy (5-fluorouracil, interferon)

The morphologic sequence from preinvasive (in situ) lesions to the early or microinvasive lesions to invasive carcinomas is frequently seen. The basaloid and bowenoid types of VIN lead to moderately to poorly differentiated squamous cell carcinomas, whereas the well-differentiated carcinoma in situ leads to the better differentiated carcinomas.

Invasive carcinoma develops multifocally in young women and usually unifocally in older patients. Most carcinomas show a border zone of more recently malignantly transformed epithelial regions. In all morphologic types of squamous cell vulvar carcinomas, the differently transformed areas can be readily distinguished (6).

Management of VIN

Treatment options and procedures for VIN are outlined in Table 13.**3**. Before any treatment option is embarked upon, preoperative colposcopy and biopsy are essential to aid decision making and plan management (9). Colposcopy is used to:

1. Define the extent of disease
2. Direct biopsies to the area of most clinically severe abnormality
3. Exclude overt invasive cancer
4. Direct, if necessary, laser treatment by visualizing anatomic landmarks, thus guiding the depth of vaporization to be determined

Conservative Management

A study of the natural history of VIN shows that there is a low risk of progression, and, indeed, there are case reports of spontaneous regression of VIN in young women. The majority of gynecologists currently treat VIN with minor procedures such as wide local excision and laser vaporization; the recurrence rate does not differ significantly with any one particular method. Young women undergoing these forms of treatment run the risk of psychosexual sequelae.

Expectant management requires long-term follow-up with biopsies as indicated and colposcopy to rule out malignancy. The patient has to be aware of this aspect of an expectant policy.

Wide Local Excision

Wide local excision with a knife or the laser is used to treat unifocal or multicentric lesions. Laser treatment is popular because it employs the unique properties of this modality, namely, removal of tissue with minimal trauma.

CO₂ Laser Vaporization

CO_2 laser vaporization treatment of VIN is associated with a recurrence rate of 5% to 40%. Recurrence is a result of ineffective treatment in either depth or lateral extent. It is possible that HPV, a known etiologic agent for VIN 3, exists in normal tissue adjacent to the lesion and as such may reinfect the healing tissue. Excellent therapeutic and cosmetic results can be obtained with laser vaporization of the hairy and nonhairy skin to depths of 2 mm and 1 mm, respectively.

Medical Therapy

Medical treatment of VIN includes chemotherapy in the forms of 5-fluorouracil dinitrochlorobenzene cream and interferon. Photodynamic therapy, involving photochemical destruction of cells sensitized with a light-activator compound such as hematoporphyrin, is undergoing trials at this time.

References

1. Wilkinson EJ, Sone IK. Atlas of vulvar disease. Baltimore: Williams & Wilkins, Baltimore 1995:1–9.
2. Friedrich EG. Vulvar disease. In: Major problems in obstetrics and gynecology. Vol. 9. Philadelphia: Saunders, 1976: 27–51.
3. Ridley CM. The vulva. Edinburgh: Churchill, 1988: 68.
4. Ridley CM, Frankman O, Jones ISC, Pincus SH, Wilkinson EJ. New nomenclature of vulvar disease. Report of the Committee on Terminology of the ISSVD. Int J Gynecol Pathol 1989;8: 83–84.
5. Ridley CM, Oriel JD, Robinson AJ. A colour atlas of diseases of the vulva. London: Chapman & Hall, London 1992:2–4.
6. Rowan RW. The natural history of vulvar intraepithelial neoplasia. Br J Obstet Gynaecol 1995;102:764–766.
7. Kaufman RH. Intraepithelial neoplasma of the vulva. Gynecol Oncol 1995;56:8–31.
8. Park JS, Jones RW, McLean MR, et al. Possible etiologic heterogeneity of vulvar intraepithelial neoplasia. Cancer 1991;67:1599–1607.
9. Singer A, Monaghan JM. Lower genital tract precancer (colposcopy, pathology and treatment). Boston: Blackwell, 1994: 177–186.

14

Subject Index

Note: Please note that as the subject of this book is colposcopy, all entries refer to this subject unless otherwise stated.